NURSING EDUCATION: Research and Developments

ERRATA

Nursing Education: Research and Developments
Edited by Bryn Davis

Page 141
line 23

Trust empathy . . .
should read
Trait empathy . . .

line 27 to 29 should read

. . . strengthened by numerous significant correlations between the Hogan Empathy Scale (trait empathy) and stable factors of personality on Cattell's 16PF test and the tendency for state empathy scores on the Empathy Construct Rating Scale.

Nursing Education: Research and Developments

Edited by Bryn Davis

CROOM HELM
London • New York • Sydney

© 1987 Bryn D. Davis

Croom Helm Ltd, Provident House, Burrell Row,
Beckenham, Kent BR3 1AT

Croom Helm Australia, 44–50 Waterloo Road,
North Ryde, 2113, New South Wales

British Library Cataloguing in Publication Data

Nursing education: research and developments.
  1. Nursing — Study and teaching
  I. Davis, Bryn D.
  610.73′07′11   RT71
  ISBN 0-7099-4508-6

Published in the USA by
Croom Helm
in association with Methuen, Inc.
29 West 35th Street
New York, NY10001

Library of Congress Cataloging-in-Publication Data

Nursing education.

  Includes index.
  1. Nursing — Study and teaching. 2. Curriculum
planning. 3. Curriculum evaluation. I. Davis, Bryn D.
[DNLM: 1. Education, Nursing. WY 18 N97873]
RT71.N776 1987   610.73′07   87-6835
ISBN 0-7099-4508-6

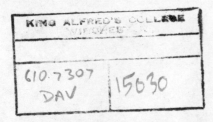
Filmset by Mayhew Typesetting, Bristol, England

Printed and bound in Great Britain by
Biddles Ltd, Guildford and King's Lynn

Contents

Acknowledgements

I would like to express my appreciation of the good spirit in which the authors of the various chapters have shared in the preparation of this volume. I feel that I have gained much from reading the various drafts and hope that the reader receives as much benefit from the final versions presented here. Tim Hardwick of Croom Helm commissioned the book in the first place and much valued editorial help and advice has been given by Christine Birdsall, also of Croom Helm, and Mary Sayers.

Bryn D. Davis
Brighton Polytechnic

Contributors

Akinsanya, J.A., BTACert, SRN, ONC, RNT, BSc, PhD, FWACN
Principal Lecturer, Department of Nursing and Community Service,
Dorset Institute of Higher Education, Poole, Dorset

Cork, N.M., SRN, HVCert, Teacher's Cert, MA
Senior Lecturer, Department of Community Studies, Brighton
Polytechnic, Falmer, Brighton, East Sussex

Cormack, D., RGN, RMN, DipEd, DipNurs, MPhil, PhD
Reader, Department of Molecular and Life Sciences, Dundee
College of Technology, Dundee, Scotland

Davis, B.D., SRN, RMN, RNT, BSc, PhD
Principal Lecturer, Department of Community Studies, Brighton
Polytechnic, Falmer, Brighton, East Sussex

Faulkner, A., SRN, RCNT, DipEd, MA, MLitt, PhD
Senior Lecturer, Department of Nursing Studies, Edinburgh University, Edinburgh, Scotland

Gallego, A.P., SRN, RNT, MA
Senior Lecturer, Department of Nursing and Community Health
Studies, Polytechnic of the Southbank, London

Jacka, K., BA
Research Associate, Nursing Education Research Unit, King's
College (London), London University, Chelsea, London

Lewin, D.C., SRN, RNT, DipEd, BA
Research Associate, Nursing Education Research Unit, King's
College (London), Chelsea, London

Macleod Clark, J., SRN, BSc, PhD
Senior Lecturer, Department of Nursing Studies, King's College
(London), Chelsea, London

McGinnis, P., RMN, DipN, Polytechnic Cert. in Personnel Skills, BSc
Director of Nursing Services (Psychiatry), Leeds

Müller, D.J., BEd, PhD, ABPsS
Professor, School of Psychology, Lancaster Polytechnic, Lancaster

Pirie, S.E.B., PGCE, MA, PhD
Lecturer, Department of Science Education, University of Warwick, Coventry

Reynolds, W., RMN, RGN, RNT, MPhil
Nurse Tutor, Highland School of Nursing, Raigmore Hospital, Inverness, Scotland

Sankar, S., SRN, RMN, RNT, BEd
Senior Tutor, School of Nursing, Cane Hill Hospital, Coulsdon, Surrey

Stapleton, M.F., RGN, SCM, DHSA, DipEd, MPhil
Nursing Officer, Special Project, DHSS, Elephant and Castle, London

Wattley, L.A., SRN, BA
Senior Lecturer, Department of Nursing and Social Studies, North East Surrey College of Technology, Epsom, Surrey

Introduction

B.D. Davis

This volume is an attempt to bring to the nursing profession a collection of reports of recent research and developments relating to nurse education. The emphasis is on research done in the UK, as in the author's previous volume (Davis, 1983). Nevertheless it is hoped that the book will be of interest to readers in other countries as well. The volume edited by Henderson (1982), for example, shows the importance of the international scene, and there is of course much research going on elsewhere. As will be shown below, however, at present nurse education in the UK is in need of research into its own particular situation.

Nurse education is at a very dynamic but uncertain stage. This uncertainty reflects a problem which has troubled the profession for many decades, that of having difficulty in making decisions on its own behalf. The uncertainty also reflects a weakness in the status of the profession which is only now beginning to be rectified. That weakness is the lack of a research base to the information required in decision-making. Instead, we have over the last few decades seen the embarrassing sight of a disunited profession, speaking with many voices, usually informed only by private experience and prejudice and rarely by scientific, professional knowledge.

However, over the last decade or so there has been the beginnings of an inroad into this professional ignorance. Research in nursing has got underway and, in particular, research into nurse education has become relatively well established. It accounts, for example, for 16 per cent of research published in *Nursing Research Abstracts* in 1985/6, the highest percentage for any of the categories of research reported. Some of this research is small scale, undertaken by nurses as part or whole requirement for higher degree studies. Other research is carried out by nurse educators as part of their work. Relatively little is carried out by teams of researchers and tackling substantial issues. Nevertheless, all of this research is adding to the sum of information becoming available to the profession. In some instances projects undertaken by individual nurses have been concerned with different aspects of the same issue and therefore combine to provide a more comprehensive picture. The areas of student nurse socialisation, and ward learning environments are cases in point (see Davis, 1983 for examples).

There have been many developments in nurse education over the last few years. These include the devolution of examinations for the register from the National Boards to schools of nursing, the introduction of new syllabuses, the attempts to implement the nursing process, the application of models of nursing to practice, a concern with learning objectives, with learning environments, clinical supervision, clinical assessment, and continuing education. Very few if any of these developments are research-based. The question of learning environments has received some attention from researchers, as has that of continuing education. The latter is only at the beginnings of being research-based, however, although the former has a relatively substantial amount of research to inform decisions.

The uncertainties and lack of cohesion in the profession as a whole can be seen in the recent publication of three separate documents proposing changes for nurse education. These were from a major professional organisation and two statutory bodies. They were published within a year of each other and offered yet more evidence of the inability of the profession to speak with a united, informed voice (ENB, 1985; RCN, 1985; UKCC, 1986).

The responses to these documents show that the majority of nurses are trying to make decisions from their private subjective knowledge base, rather than from an informed academic base. It is to be hoped that decisions made with respect to the future of nurse education at this time are not taken out of the hands of nurses, nor are made without reference to the growing body of evidence available from within the profession and from elsewhere.

RECENT RESEARCH

In reviewing the recent British literature on research, development and writing about nurse education, a wide range of material was identified. Some of this work is completed and published as articles in nursing journals. Others are still ongoing and are referred to in *Abstracts of Nursing Research*, published by the DHSS.

Rogers (1985) has identified five areas of priority in nursing education research. These are curriculum content; methods of teaching and learning; the assessment of learners; the preparation of the nurse teacher; and models for nurse education. Her view of these priorities was derived from a review of the literature published mainly in the early 1980s.

Looking at the literature published or reported since then, it would seem that these priorities have been adhered to in the choice of topics in nurse education research. The majority of projects have been concerned with methods of teaching and the clinical learning environment. The latter group of projects have looked in part at the preparation of ward staff for their teaching/supervisor role. The former group have involved a wide variety of teaching strategies, including skills analysis, experiential learning, syndicate learning, learning through incidents, and various aspects of student-centred inquiry methods. Several projects were concerned with the use of computers.

A large proportion of reports involve issues in curriculum content, a majority of these studying aspects of post-basic education. However, relatively few projects have studied the assessment of learners or models in curriculum development, although there continues to be a major interest in student nurse socialisation.

Another major area of interest, not identified by Rogers, has been that of evaluation of nurse education, with projects looking at sections of the curriculum, the whole curriculum, various clinical experiences as part of a curriculum, and whole schools of nursing.

These categories of research reflect a process approach to nursing education, advocated by Davis (1983) supported by Rogers (1985) and reflected in the more recent literature. That is, they show a concern with the assessment of learners' needs (curriculum content); the planning and implementation of curricula (models of education: methods of teaching and the provision of learning environments); and evaluation (student assessment: curriculum and school evaluation).

A SELECTION OF RESEARCH

This book attempts to make available to the nursing profession examples of recent research in order that the current practice may be as well informed as possible and also so that those making decisions about the future of nursing education do so on the best possible evidence. Part I looks at what to teach nurses; Part II looks at how to teach various subjects to nurses; and Part III has chapters on the evaluation of the educational process.

The first chapter involves a review by Morwenna Cork of approaches to curriculum planning. This takes principles from general education and shows how they can be applied to nurse education. Various models are considered and discussed to help the nurse educationalist in making decisions about curriculum development. This chapter plays a scene-setting role for the rest of the volume.

The question of what to teach nurses is a major factor in making decisions about curriculum development and the next three chapters deal with this issue. Justus Akinsanya has already made a name for himself in arguing the case for a strong basis of biological sciences in nurse education. Here he reports a survey of course directors, nurse tutors and learners as to their views and practices regarding the subject. He then uses this evidence to suggest future developments. Susan Pirie, as a mathematician, has been concerned about the numeracy of nurses and what aspects of mathematics should be taught to them. She reports her research into the levels of numeracy needed by nurses, presents a taxonomy of mathematics for nursing and discusses the implications for nurse education. Finally, Mary Stapleton gives us the results of her study of post-basic education needs perceived by trained nurses, and their satisfaction with current provisions. Her argument is that without such information the work of those involved in post-basic nurse education is more likely to be a hit-and-miss affair.

There then follow a series of chapters on how to teach nurses. Many of these are concerned with aspects of communication and interpersonal skills in various professional settings. Three also refer to psychiatric nursing. This is a further example of how different researchers can complement each other. The first chapter is by Bill Reynolds and Desmond Cormack and concerns the integration of theory and practice. Their research involves the teaching of interpersonal skills in the clinical setting and utilising a student-centred approach. They discuss in some detail different models of nursing that can be applied, considering the role of the psychiatric nurse and the place of interpersonal skills in the therapeutic relationship. The chapter by Sandy Sankar concerns the application of a particular model of nursing to the psychiatric setting and shows how principles of curriculum development can be related to a model of nursing to produce a relevant basis for nurse education. The chapter reports a pilot study undertaken to demonstrate the process, with reference to the teaching of interpersonal skills in the introductory course. The author highlights difficulties and suggests developments.

The other chapters in this section involve psychology for nurses, teaching communication skills and teaching nurses to teach. Lesley Wattley and Dave Müller have written elsewhere in some detail about their approach to the teaching of psychology to nurses. In their chapter they summarise their case for an experiential approach and offer some examples for nurse tutors wishing to take up their ideas. Jill Macleod Clark and Ann Faulkner report on the outcome of a nationwide survey undertaken with the support of the Health Education Council into the teaching of communication skills to nurses. They show a very revealing picture of the attitudes and practice of DNEs, nurse tutors and learners and offer suggestions for future developments, including workshops to facilitate change in this area. Finally, Peter McGinnis describes his approach to the preparation of nurses for an educational role in their practice. Drawing on evidence indicating the importance of the nurse being able to teach the patient, and co-ordinating models of nursing and education, he provides nurse educators with information to help them prepare their own strategies.

The final section of this book contains two chapters offering information about the evaluation of nurse education. The first, by Amalia Gallego, reports her research into the evaluation of a school of nursing. In this she discusses the nature of evaluation, the criteria that can be used, and in her single case-study demonstrates the types of evaluation that are possible. She makes an interesting and valuable comparison between methods of course approval and evaluation in nursing and higher education. The other chapter in this section, by David Lewin and Keith Jacka, looks at the evaluation of the uptake of educational opportunities for the application in practice of theoretical input by student nurses. They demonstrate a relatively simple method that could be applied in any school.

The authors of each chapter provide a reference list which should enable others to investigate further the particular issues raised.

CONCLUSION

In the light of the present dynamic and uncertain situation regarding the future of nursing education, there is an urgent need to focus research in a way that will help the profession to answer questions and resolve that uncertainty. This would seem to imply much more evidence relating to models of education applied to nursing in order to achieve the outcome of an assessing, planning, implementing, and evaluating approach to nursing patients who are seen as whole people. There is also an equivalent need for research into the content of suitable curricula to meet the students' needs, including the level of content as well as the type. Associated with this issue is that of the relation between theory and practice and the development of the optimum strategies for the effective integration of the two. In this way nurses should then be informed in their assessment of need and delivery of care, and able to justify it to others. This necessitates links between and the co-ordination of models of nursing and models of education (see Davis, 1986, for a review of current books in print on this topic). Finally, more research is required into the nature of and preparation for nurse teaching, clinical facilitation and supervision of practice, although this is an area where a beginning is being made.

In many ways there is a confusing relationship between research and development in nursing. Sometimes developments occur without planned preparatory work, including research. As a profession we have not been able to take advantage of such changes and use them to provide reliable and valid information. Consequently there has been little learning from experience, particularly as many of the developments affecting nursing have been imposed by other agencies. Now, however, with the beginnings of a research base we are more able to anticipate change or to use change as a focus for our research efforts.

In the present climate, with the nursing profession actually proposing or even demanding changes, it is most important that we speak with an informed voice, and as far as possible have the support of previous and current research findings for our arguments. Even if the findings currently available do not provide all the answers needed, a high profile of relevant research activity will increase the professional status of nursing, and will strengthen the hands of those speaking for us around negotiating tables. A profession that knows how, why and where it wants to go is much more likely to get there.

REFERENCES

Davis, B.D. (1983) *Research into nurse education*. Croom Helm, London

Davis, B.D. (1986) Nurse education, *British Book News*, May, 275–8

ENB (1985) *Professional education/training courses. Consultation Paper*. English National Board for Nursing, Midwifery and Health Visiting, London

Henderson, M.S. (1982) *Recent advances in nursing: education*. Churchill Livingstone, Edinburgh

RCN (1985) The education of nurses: a new dispensation, *Commision on Nursing Education*. Royal College of Nursing of the United Kingdom, London

Rogers, J.M. (1985) An examination of research priorities in nurse education, *Journal of Advanced Nursing*, *10*, 233–6

UKCC (1986) *Project 2000: a new preparation for practice*. United Kingdom Central Council for Nursing, Midwifery and Health Visiting, London

1

Approaches to Curriculum Planning

N.M. Cork

INTRODUCTION

Over recent years the study of the curriculum has assumed increasing importance in all fields of education. For nurse educators the significance of such study is of vital concern. By its very nature, nurse education is a complex mixture of theory drawn from different disciplines, and practised in a variety of care settings. It is therefore essential that those involved in the development of nursing curricula have a knowledge and understanding of the principles of curriculum planning in order to create a coherent, structured and comprehensive learning programme. Such a programme should not only enable the students to attain the competencies laid down by the English National Board for Nursing, Midwifery and Heath Visiting (ENB) but should also develop their intellectual skills so that they may continue to learn throughout their careers.

Initial nurse training is, as the name implies, only the beginning of learning to nurse. The professional nurse must accept a responsibility for continued learning, both informally and formally through attendance on courses. Similarly the profession as a whole must recognise the importance of post-basic education and the need to fund nurses to attend such courses. Mary Stapleton has discussed this issue more fully in her chapter on post-basic education needs (Chapter 4).

Whether one is concerned with the development of initial nurse education courses or of post-basic courses, the principles of curriculum planning are of relevance. In this chapter I intend to look at some of the key issues in the planning process from the inception of an idea, through decisions on content and structure, the use of curriculum models, and problems of achieving integration in the curriculum, and finally to the evaluation of the curriculum.

DEFINING THE CURRICULUM

Any discussion of curriculum planning must commence with a review of definitions of the curriculum. One of the most well known definitions is that given by Stenhouse (1975): 'A curriculum is an attempt to communicate the essential principles and features of an educational proposal in such a form that it is open to critical scrutiny and capable of effective translation into practice' (p. 4). This definition implies that a curriculum is produced in a written or visual form for examination by others. It may sometimes appear that the main purpose of the documentation of the curriculum is for validation of a course. However, Stenhouse does go on to emphasise that the course as presented should be feasible in practice. This is an important point as it is very easy in curriculum planning to get bound up in the production of an academic document that bears little relation to what can actually be achieved in practice.

Kerr (1968) defines the curriculum as: 'All the learning activities which are planned and guided by the school, whether they are carried out in groups or individually, inside and outside the school' (p. 16). This definition is important as it reminds us that in nurse education/training, much of the learning will take place in the various care settings, be it a medical ward, accident and emergency department or community experience. Also the student may receive teaching on a one-to-one basis — particularly in relation to the development of practical skills, in small groups in the clinical and school setting, or in large groups in the formal lecture-room setting. It must also be recognised that some of the learning activities will be the responsibility of 'non-teaching' staff. Kerr's definition emphasises that even though learning takes place in other settings, this learning must be *planned and guided* by the school, and therefore this learning is an integral part of the curriculum.

In relation to nursing Bevis (1982) states: 'The curriculum is the manifestation of many composite parts and factors which together enable the achievement of nursing educational goals that have been fully identified, selected and articulated' (p. 8). The question of the identification, selection and articulation of educational goals is fundamental to the process of curriculum planning, and is one of the areas that calls for detailed debate. The goals determined will have an influence on content, teaching methods and assessment, all of which will be documented within the curriculum.

Quinn (1980) looks at the way the concept of the curriculum has been subdivided, and considers the relevance to nursing of these

2

sub-categories:

> official curriculum — the one laid down by the policy of the school;
> actual curriculum — the one which is taught by the teacher;
> formal curriculum — all learning which is planned by the school;
> hidden curriculum — the attitudes and values which are transmitted by the hospital (p. 73)

The official curriculum and the formal curriculum may be documented, but the actual curriculum may be at variance with the documentation, either because of constraints that become apparent as attempts are made to implement the official curriculum, or because of a need to respond quickly to the needs of the learners or to changes in local and national policies.

The hidden curriculum presents a more complex and problematic perspective. It is important that the school recognises that attitudes and values of staff in the clinical setting will impinge upon the students, and in extreme cases may cause personal conflict as the student tries to reconcile two opposing sets of values. However, the extent to which the 'hidden curriculum' can be controlled or taken account of in the planning process is variable. Certainly some opportunity can be provided for group discussions on the gulf between theory and practice: it is interesting to note that students on degree courses in nursing, although they perceive a much wider gulf between the two, actually experience less anxiety in relation to this because thay have been prepared for the discrepancy by their lecturers (Cork, 1986). Another approach to dealing with the 'hidden curriculum' is through the ongoing education of practitioners so that the values of the tutors and the values of the practitioners become more closely aligned, as Barnett, Becher and Cork (1986) suggest:

> [Tutors] must also be prepared to give substantial attention to continuing professional education if they are to create a climate among practitioners which is conducive to their assuming a major role in practical teaching. They must seek to create not only a set of shared values but also a substantial reduction in the social distance which is normally found between academics and practitioners in any professional field. (p. 24)

INNOVATION IN THE CURRICULUM

Having considered what is meant by curriculum, the next step is to look at how curriculum change may be brought about. In 1985 two major reports on nurse education (Commission on Nursing Education, 1985; ENB, 1985) were published. Both reports emphasise the need for nurse training to become much more of an educational experience for students, whether that experience be under the auspices of the health authority or the education authority (Dufton, 1985). In order to create an educational rather than a training course there will need to be profound changes in the curriculum. For such change to take place there must first be an acceptance of the new ideas by key people within the community. Havelock (1973), when discussing ways of getting an innovation accepted by others, says:

> Diffusion of an innovation begins with the acceptance of the idea by a few key members of a community. From there on it begins to spread more rapidly, usually through word-of-mouth . . . This person-to-person process is very effective; once it has started and there are clusters of people who accept the idea and who are 'talking it up' it gathers momentum. (p. 114)

He draws attention to three groups of people who play a significant part in getting the innovation accepted. They are the 'innovators', the 'leaders' and the 'resisters'. The innovator is by definition the first person to take up a new idea and is generally from within the institution; he or she is thus an 'insider'. The leader may be an 'opinion leader' who is held in high esteem and whose ideas are valued; he may be an 'insider' or from outside the institution — an 'outsider'. Another type of leader may be a 'formal leader' who holds a position of authority within the institution and has access to power coercive strategies to force change. The leader may be a 'gate-keeper' who has control over access both to people and to resources in the user system. The 'resisters' are those who critically question the innovation and may attempt to prevent or delay its implementation. They have a valuable role to play in ensuring that an innovation is not adopted too hastily and without due consideration of its full implications.

If new nursing curricula are to be implemented in relation either to initial nurse training or to post-basic courses, then those members within schools of nursing or institutions of higher education who wish to introduce change will need to negotiate with colleagues and other interested parties, for example staff in the clinical setting, to get the change accepted. Bennis, Benne and Chinn (1969) discuss three types of strategies that people may use when negotiating change.[1] The first they refer to as empirical–rational strategies. They state that the assumptions underlying these strategies are: 'that men are rational . . . that men will follow their rational self-interest once this is revealed to them'. This approach involves highlighting and emphasising the advantages to be gained by the proposed change and possibly backing this up with supporting evidence from research.

The second approach is through normative–reeducative strategies. The assumptions underlying this are: 'Patterns of action and practice are supported by socio-cultural norms and by commitments on the part of the individual to these norms. Socio-cultural norms are supported by the attitude and value systems of individuals.' To bring about change through this approach requires not merely that the individual accepts change but that there is a fundamental shift in his or her attitude and values so that change is viewed as consistent with his or her socio-cultural norms.

The third approach discussed by Bennis *et al.* is a power coercive strategy. Of this strategy they say: 'In general, emphasis is upon political and economic sanctions in the exercise of power. But other coercive strategies emphasise the utilization of moral power, playing upon sentiments of guilt and shame.' Using this approach people may be forced to accept change because the person who wishes to initiate change is in a position to exert control over them through, for example, the use of rewards and punishments.

Hoyle (1972) identified five significant dimensions to change: the rate of change, the scale of change, the degree of change, the continuity of change, and the direction of change. The extent to which each of these is relevant will depend on whether the proposed innovation relates to the broad spectrum of nurse training or to one specific aspect of an initial or post-basic course. As a whole, nursing at present seems to be in a period of rapid change; the scale of the proposed change in initial nurse training is vast and the degree to which such a change will affect nursing is profound in that it is a fundamental change from a training to an educational course. In that the current changes stem from change proposed in the Briggs Report (1972), these changes may be seen as a process of evolution rather than revolution.

In order, then, for change to be implemented and new curricula to be developed, there first needs to be the adoption of a new idea

Figure 1.1: From innovation to adoption

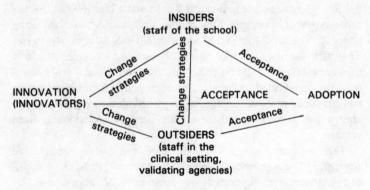

by key people, the innovators, and there needs to be negotiation with all members of the school and relevant outside bodies to promote acceptance and thus adoption of the new scheme. Quinn (1980) stresses the importance of open discussion between staff of the school if innovation is to be viewed positively, emphasising that innovation may have greater acceptability if it stems from within the organization, particularly if it is seen as responsive in terms of curriculum evaluation and in line with the values of the course team. With regard to nursing it is also important to recognise that for full adoption of a new idea there must also be negotiation with outsiders including practitioners and validation agencies. This process of adoption is illustrated in Figure 1.1. As Figure 1.1 indicates, not only may the 'insiders' and the 'outsiders' be required to change their perspective, but also the innovator may be required to modify his or her original ideas in order to gain their acceptance and adoption in practice.

THE PROCESS OF CURRICULUM PLANNING

Literature on curriculum development stresses the importance of a logical step-by-step approach to curriculum planning (Taba, 1962; Stenhouse, 1975; Pratt, 1980; Rowntree, 1981; Bevis, 1982; Kelly, 1982; Lee and Zeldin, 1982; Torres and Stanton, 1982). For the majority the planning process is seen to consist of four main elements. Taba (1962) considers these elements to be: a statement of aims and objectives; the selection and organisation of content; the patterns of teaching and learning; and a programme of evaluation of

Figure 1.2: Basic curriculum model

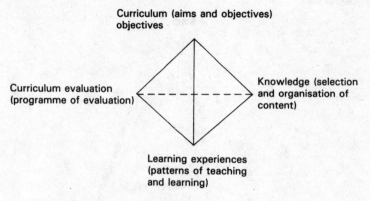

Source: modified from Kerr, 1968, p. 17.

the outcome (p. 10). These elements in fact form the basis of many curriculum models, including Kerr's 'simple model of the curriculum' (Kerr, 1968, p. 17). This model and Taba's four elements are shown in Figure 1.2. This basic model may stimulate some initial thoughts on the organisation of the curriculum, but there are other aspects which may be added to present a more complete picture of factors to be considered when planning nursing curricula. The model given by Eraut (1976) adds important dimensions which are of significance to nurse educators (Figure 1.3). This model focuses on the relationship between aims and curriculum decisions, and Eraut suggests:

> . . . an emphasis on knowledge leads to early decisions on Subject Matter; an emphasis on skills to an analysis of Objectives; an emphasis on certification or selection to a concern for Assessment and an emphasis on attitudes and relationships to a consideration of Teaching and Learning. (p. 20)

Eraut's model is useful in that it highlights the fact that decisions in any one area will influence and possibly constrain decisions in other areas. Thus decisions on the range and quantity of subject matter will influence choice of teaching methods and assessment procedures. The formulated objectives will in turn guide the approaches to teaching and assessment, and may constrain the choice of subject matter.

Figure 1.3: The relationship between aims and curriculum decisions

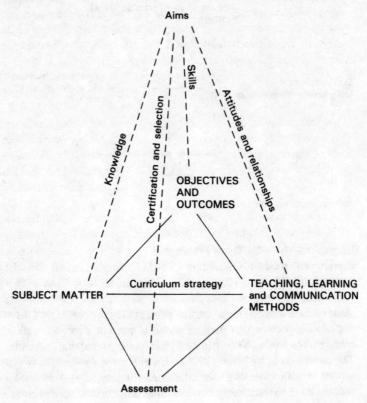

Source: Eraut (1976).

The components of the model also draw attention to the fact that in some areas decisions are going to be strongly affected by external factors. The issue of qualification and classification is of increasing importance to nurse educators in the light of recent recommendations to foster the development of initial nurse education under the auspices of local colleges or polytechnics. There will be a need to satisfy the ENB that courses provide the theoretical and practical experience necessary to develop the students' competence in order that they may receive the professional qualification. Demands may also be made from within the institution and from external validating bodies such as the Council for National Academic Awards if courses are to be classified as certificate, diploma or degree courses. Recommendations and directives from validating bodies may strongly influence the choice and range of subject matter and the assessment procedures. For example, in relation to degree courses it may be the nature of the students' final dissertation which decides whether the course is deemed to be an honours degree course or not.

An acknowledgement of constraints is an important early step in the curriculum planning process. Pratt (1980) says of constraints:

A constraint is a factor external to a system that limits the capability of the system . . . some of the constraints that frequently influence the design of the curriculum are the learners, politics, policy, external examinations, financial and material limitations, staffing, time and the physical environment. (p. 110)

It is worth considering each of these constraints individually as it will help to highlight some important issues to which curriculum planners need to give attention.

The learners' anticipated knowledge base needs to be considered because of its implications for the level at which lecturers/tutors should direct their teaching and the content of syllabuses. The age range of students may also be significant as age is a significant factor in adaptation to learning (Knowles, 1970; Mezirow, 1983; Birchenall, 1985). Previous experience may also need to be taken into account, particularly on post-registration courses where some students may only have their basic nursing qualification whereas others may have midwifery, district nursing or health visiting qualifications.

Politics in relation to nurse education may be significant at government level in that recommendations and directives may be given on education and training in reports and government papers. Of note is the recent report on community nursing (DHSS, 1986a), which included recommendations of significance to the training of health visitors, district nurses and school nurses, and the Green Paper on primary health care (DHSS, 1986b). The publication of Project 2000, the report on the education and training of nurses, will potentially exert a very strong influence on nursing curricula. Politics may also be significant at a local level in relation to the siting of courses and the potential involvement of different institutions in providing experience for students.

Policy issues, such as internal and external validation procedures, may be relevant. In addition the policy of the school of nursing may

9

affect the size of the student group and the potential for staff to attend courses, which in turn may affect their willingness to take on new areas of responsibility and the role relationships between staff in the school and staff in the clinical setting.

External examinations are becoming less important as examinations and assessment procedures are increasingly internally controlled. However, the role of the validating agencies, as previously mentioned, is very significant, and they may well constrain the choice of objectives, subject matter and assessment.

Financial and material limitations may be significant in deciding upon the teaching methods to be used, the range of experience to be provided and the availability of library and media resources. For example, it may be considered that the teaching of communication and interpersonal skills may be facilitated by the use of interactive video (whether this is an option or not will depend on resources). Similarly the potential for students to gain from self-directed study will be influenced by the library and media resources available to them.

Staffing levels have implications for choice of teaching method and for the potential for small group work and one-to-one teaching. The opportunity for staff to develop expertise in one area is also influenced by staffing levels. Where student–staff ratios are high, staff may be expected to cover a wide range of teaching topics and have little time to study one area in depth. The other important issue as regards staffing is an acknowledgement of the difficulties of staff from the school in guiding and directing the students' learning in the clinical setting.

Time may be a very severe constraint on curriculum planning as the time scale for developing new courses or revising existing ones may be limited. It is also necessary to recognise that course development generally has to take place alongside all other work and can thus substantially increase the individual's work load.

Physical environment is particularly important with regard to nurse training because of the different clinical settings that may need to be used. This may be a severe constraint as regards staff of the school working with students in these clinical settings.

Evans (1982) also gives an interesting summary of the factors that may influence nursing curricula. He identifies two main spheres of influence; teacher-centred influences which include education-service issues, teacher expertise, student abilities and examinations; and resource-centred influences, including political, physical and clinical resources.

Figure 1.4: Hoy and Mustafa's (1983) curriculum model

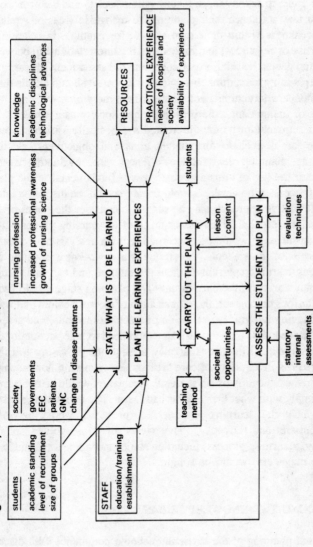

Source: Hoy and Mustafa (1983).

Hoy and Mustafa (1983) present a useful curriculum model, which highlights the factors to be taken into account when planning nursing curricula. This is given in Figure 1.4. An examination of a model such as this will help curriculum planners to identify constraints; to acknowledge factors within society and the profession which may influence their planning; to recognise areas of strength and weakness within their own school, for example in relation to expertise or resources; and to focus on the interrelationship between learning needs, learning experiences and the assessment of learning. If the planning team think through each aspect, it should enable them to produce a structured, coherent programme which will meet the needs of the students, the profession and society as a whole.

The curriculum models presented are basically variations on a theme, as all include formulating aims and objectives, selecting content, planning learning experiences and evaluating these. Whether the use of aims and objectives is fundamental to the planning process is, however, open to debate, as will be discussed later. An alternative approach may be simply to consider the stages of the curriculum process as similar to those of the nursing process. The assessment stage would be concerned with an analysis of the learning needs of the students, the strengths and weaknesses within the teaching/learning environment and the internal and external factors that may constrain the curriculum. The planning stage would focus on decisions on content, the organisation of the curriculum and ways of achieving integration, selection of teaching methods, and assessment procedures. Implementation would need to take account of the organisational difficulties that may arise from providing learning experiences in a variety of care settings and involving non-teaching staff in the education of the students. Evaluation would be concerned not simply with what the students had learnt, but also with the extent to which the learning experiences provided were the most appropriate and effective. The views of all involved in the teaching/learning process, including students, tutors, ward staff and nurse managers, would be sought.

DEFINING THE KNOWLEDGE BASE

Detailed planning of the curriculum should commence with discussions of what the students need to learn. This may lead to a debate about the extrinsic and intrinsic value of knowledge. Guba and Lincoln (1981) suggest that:

There are two senses in which an entity may have value. On the one hand it may have value of its own, implicit, inherent, independent of any possible applications . . . we shall apply the term *merit* to this kind of intrinsic, context-free value. On the other hand an entity may have value within some context of use or application . . . we shall apply the term *worth* to this kind of extrinsic or context-determined value. (p. 39)

Historically many nursing curricula have emphasised the extrinsic value of the knowledge to be transmitted in terms of its direct worth within the nursing context. There are, however, many reasons for developing curricula that allow for the inclusion of areas of knowledge which are of intrinsic value. For example, in relation to the study of disciplines such as sociology and psychology, students need to develop an understanding of the basic concepts, theories and principles of procedure fundamental to the discipline, not simply those aspects applicable to nursing. Such a fundamental understanding of the disciplines should help to foster powers of logic and critical thought (Peters, 1966, 1977; Hirst, 1974; Stenhouse, 1975), and should facilitate the students' personal development.

Such an approach is also important if learning to nurse is to be an educational experience, not simply a form of training. In its most basic form, training is generally held to be the inculcation of a specific skill, requiring set behavioural responses, often without reference to the general principles underlying the skill. Thus a person may be trained to carry out a specific task and yet have no understanding of the significance of the required behavioural pattern. As Paterson (1979) says:

What essentially differentiates a process of training from a process of education is this deliberate restriction and compression of the trainee's awareness, which is focussed tightly on some comparatively limited set of operations, temporarily disconnected from their wider cognitive setting. (p. 288)

Education, on the other hand, is concerned with giving people a body of knowledge and awareness of basic principles that helps them to develop a conceptual framework on which they can build in the future (Peters, 1967; Paterson, 1979).

The emphasis in nursing has shifted in recent years from training to education. Much of the impetus for this has stemmed from the move from a focus on the task to a focus on the individual, as

13

Sheahan (1980) says:

> Nursing practice and thus the teaching of nursing practice has
> been given a new direction in recent years with the introduction
> of the nursing process. This change of direction has been from
> a task-centred approach to a person-centred approach. Among the
> claims made for the nursing process, apart from its individualistic
> orientation, is that it is a scientific, an analytical, a rational and
> a problem-solving approach to the delivery of nursing care.
> (p. 494)

The use of the nursing process is generally held to improve the
quality of nursing care (Little and Carnevali, 1976; Johnston, 1978;
Kratz, 1979; Gott, 1982). The term 'quality nursing care' may be
used to differentiate between safe nursing practice and optimum
nursing practice. A nurse may be technically competent to carry out
a specific nursing procedure but may do so in a mechanistic way
which almost ignores the presence of the patient except as an object
to be acted upon. With quality nursing care there is respect for the
individual as a rational thinking human being and an active participant in the health-care process. It involves an awareness of the right
of the patient to information and an honest explanation of the
procedures that are to be carried out. During any patient/nurse
interaction there must be communication which conveys a sensitivity
to the patient's needs and acknowledges his worth as an individual.
As Smith (1982) states: 'Thus quality nursing care incorporates
interpersonal and communication skills with technical expertise and
knowledge to minimise patient anxiety and discomfort' (p. 119).

The concept of total patient care is of particular significance
because of its impact on the content of the curriculum. The acceptance of man as a biopsychosocial being (Rogers, 1970; King, 1971;
Roy, 1976) and the need for a holistic approach to nursing care will
lead to the inclusion of social and behavioural sciences and an
emphasis on the integration of these disciplines with the biological
sciences.

A key factor which should guide the curriculum planners is also
their view of what the end product of the course should be like. This
point is emphasised by Smith (1982):

> It is also to be argued that in order to generate and structure nurs-
> ing knowledge, a conceptualization of the nurse and nursing is
> required to prove guidance in curriculum development and

empirical study. In addition it is thought necessary that a nursing faculty achieve consensus regarding their publicly stated conceptualization of a nurse and nursing so that the curriculum is, at once, presented and experienced as a unified whole. (p. 117)

She goes on to discuss the implications that the agreed conceptualisation of a nurse has for the way in which the curriculum is designed, the content of the course and the teaching strategies employed. For example, if the conceptualisation of a nurse includes a problem-solving approach to her work, this can be negated if the teaching strategies used are very didactic and allow no opportunity for experiential learning.

Linked to the conceptualisation of the nurse is the use of models of nursing to provide a conceptual framework of nursing and thus a frame of reference for the curriculum planner (Henderson, 1978; Meleis, 1979; Brown and Lee, 1980; McFarlane, 1980; Smith, 1982; Collister, 1983; Arthurs, 1984; Chapman, 1984; Roberts, 1985). Where a school elects to use a specific nursing model as a focus for curriculum planning, the model selected will influence content, learning experiences, teaching method and assessment (Stevens, 1979; Riehl and Roy, 1980; Smith, 1982; Roper, Logan and Tierney, 1983; Arthurs, 1984). For example, where a school selects Orem's self-care nursing model (Orem, 1980), there will be a need to focus on health rather than ill-health, self-care behaviour as the coping mechanism in the event of ill-health, and nursing interventions to promote self-care. Learning experiences and teaching methods must foster communication and interpersonal skills and in particular teaching skills in order that the nurse may promote the individual's ability to engage in self-care. Similarly, as Smith (1982) says: 'If Roy's (1976) model is selected then the four adaptive modes, physiologic needs, self-concept, role function and interdependence are fundamental to the development of any nursing course based on this model' (p. 121).

McGlynn (1984) sees the nursing model as the medium through which nursing theory may direct nursing practice. He states:

A model may be defined as a symbolic representation of an idealised situation; it is a conception of reality, never reality itself. Nursing models are abstractions based upon scientifically identified concepts and theories central to nursing; they are idealised representations of reality . . . Valid nursing theory directs nursing practice through the medium of a nursing model or models. (p. 47)

15

The potential use of a model of nursing for curriculum planning needs to be considered by the course team. It should at the very least generate a useful debate on the nature of nursing and nursing knowledge which will help the team in the formulation of the aims and objectives for the course. The complexities of organising a curriculum around a model of nursing should, however, be acknowledged. It requires an in-depth knowledge of the model selected and an ability to see how the disciplines interrelate to provide the structure for the analysis of nursing through the given model. In many colleges and schools of nursing, aspects of the curriculum may be dealt with by lecturers who have a discipline base and an understanding of the relevance and application of the discipline to nursing. Their knowledge, however, may not be sufficient for them to effectively use a model of nursing as the tool for abstracting the essentials of the discipline of relevance to nursing, or as the basis for the analysis of the key concepts of the discipline. It may in fact be argued that to structure the curriculum around a model of nursing would provide too narrow a focus for the contributory disciplines, and students would not develop the basic understanding of the disciplines necessary for ongoing learning.

APPROACHES TO CURRICULUM PLANNING

The most well documented approach to curriculum planning is undoubtedly through the use of objectives, as noted by Tyler (1949) who said:

> Since the real purpose of education is . . . to bring about significant changes in the student's pattern of behaviour, it becomes important to recognise that any statement of objectives of the school should be a statement of changes to take place in the student. (in Lee and Zeldin, 1982, p. 160)

by Taba (1962):

> Educational objectives have a variety of functions. Perhaps the most important one is that of guiding decisions about the selection of content and of learning experiences and of providing criteria on what to teach and how to teach it. (p. 197)

and by Torres and Stanton (1982), who look at the importance of providing objectives for each year of the student's programme. They refer to these as level objectives and state:

> Level objectives are derived from the characteristics of the graduate and are reflective of the theoretical framework. They make explicit an expected change in the learner at an identified point in time within the total programme which allows for cumulative learning. (p. 60)

Davies (1976), in his discussion of the use of objectives in curriculum design, differentiates between aims, goals or general objectives and specific or behavioural objectives. He says:

> An aim can broadly be defined as a general statement, which attempts to give both shape and direction to a set of more detailed intentions for the future . . . Aims play an important role in making explicit and public those activities that we finally regarded as being educationally valuable and worthwhile. . . . general objectives respresent an attempt to operationalise the thinking represented by an aim to make it more practical and less ethereal . . . Specific objectives attempt to describe, in the clearest terms possible, exactly what a student will think, act or feel at the end of a learning experience. (pp. 12–15)

The need to differentiate between aims and objectives is also discussed by Sheahan (1978) and Quinn (1980). Whereas aims may be fairly broad and reflect the philosophy of the course, the objectives must be much more specific and capable of measurement. It is generally considered that a well formulated objective will state clearly the behaviour to be demonstrated, the range of acceptable behaviour, the context in which the behaviour may be demonstrated and any special conditions relevant to the performance of the behaviour.

Because of the complexity of formulating objectives and the recognition that learning did not simply relate to the acquisition of knowledge, Benjamin Bloom and colleagues in 1948 set out to draw up a taxonomy of educational objectives. They identified three major spheres of learning, the first related to knowledge and intellectual functioning, which they referred to as the cognitive domain, the second related to attitudes, values and feelings, this being referred to as the affective domain, and the last related to the development of motor skills, the psychomotor domain (Bloom, 1956). The

17

Table 1.1: Taxonomies for educational objectives

Level	Cognitive domain (Bloom, 1956)	Affective domain (Krathwohl, 1964)	Psychomotor domain (Harrow, 1972)	Psychomotor domain (Simpson, 1972)
1.00	Knowledge	Receiving	Reflex movement	Perception
2.00	Comprehension	Responding	Basic fundamental movements	Set
3.00	Application	Valuing	Perceptual abilities	Guided response
4.00	Analysis	Organisation	Physical abilities	Mechanism
5.00	Synthesis	Characterisation	Skilled movements	Complex overt response
6.00	Evaluation		Non-discursive communication	Adaptation
7.00				Origination

taxonomies produced for each domain identify levels of behaviour moving from basic to complex responses. Table 1.1 gives these levels for each domain.

A more detailed breakdown of each domain, examples of associated action verbs which may be used when writing objectives, and some examples of objectives are given in Davies (1976), pp. 147–64. Some very useful examples of nursing objectives in relation to the cognitive and affective domain are given in Quinn (1980), pp. 89–91. Redman (1984) also gives concrete examples of nursing objectives related to the educational role of the nurse. Taba (1962), when discussing the use of objectives, identifies four levels of knowledge to which the objectives may be directed. These are given in Figure 1.5.

Figure 1.5: Levels of knowledge

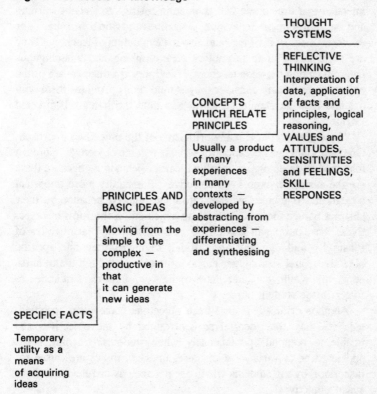

THOUGHT
SYSTEMS

REFLECTIVE
THINKING
Interpretation of
data, application
of facts and
principles, logical
reasoning,
VALUES and
ATTITUDES,
SENSITIVITIES
and FEELINGS,
SKILL
RESPONSES

CONCEPTS
WHICH RELATE
PRINCIPLES

Usually a product
of many
experiences
in many
contexts —
developed by
abstracting from
experiences —
differentiating
and synthesising

PRINCIPLES AND
BASIC IDEAS

Moving from the
simple to the
complex —
productive in
that
it can generate
new ideas

SPECIFIC FACTS

Temporary
utility as a
means
of acquiring
ideas

Source: Adapted from Taba (1962), pp. 211–28

This model can again provide a useful guide to the drawing up of objectives for a nursing curriculum and more specifically for subject areas within the curriculum. The level of knowledge to be focused on will depend on the stage of the course the student has reached and may also vary with the discipline being studied. For example, in relation to physiology and pharmacology the emphasis may be on specific facts, principles and basic ideas; and thought systems may focus on interpretation of data and the application of facts and principles. In contrast, when studying the disciplines of psychology and sociology the emphasis may be on principles and basic ideas and on concepts that relate principles, and thought systems may focus on reflective thinking, logical reasoning, and values and attitudes.

The value of an objective approach is often held to lie in the way it demands that curriculum planners clearly articulate what it is intended that the course will achieve in relation to student learning and thus subsequent behaviour. Objectives provide a firm basis for the assessment of learning, and also the evaluation of teaching. They are seen as useful in promoting clear thinking and unambiguous communication between teachers. If learners are made aware of the objectives, as many consider they should be, it provides them with a guide to what should be learnt and thus facilitates self-directed learning.

There are of course many criticisms of the objectives approach. One important consideration for some is that the objectives approach may lead to an emphasis on trivial learner behaviours because these are the easiest to express as objectives. Potentially more important educational outcomes will therefore be ignored because by their abstract nature they are difficult to articulate in the form of objectives. An example in relation to nursing may be that qualities of sensitivity and empathy are difficult to incorporate into specific objectives, and so may get pushed to one side though many nurse educators would consider them to be very important qualities to foster in the student nurse.

Another criticism is that once objectives have been specified, teachers may find themselves constrained by the objectives and unable to respond spontaneously when students' learning needs appear to be at variance with these, or when topics are raised for discussion by the students which are not seen as of relevance to the stated objectives.

One major criticism is the difficulty in formulating meaningful objectives in relation to all learning experiences. Many in the field of education consider the formulation of objectives to be a time-consuming academic exercise of little value in relation to the every-day world of the teacher.

The objectives approach has also been criticised because, as Popham (1968) notes, 'It is somehow undemocratic to plan in advance precisely how the learner should behave after instruction.' There is in fact concern that, taken to extreme, an objectives approach will result in all learners exhibiting identical behaviours and being unable to go beyond the prescribed behaviour (Stenhouse, 1975).

An alternative approach to curriculum design has been proposed by Stenhouse (1975). He suggests that:

> Within knowledge and arts areas it is possible to select content for a curriculum unit without reference to student behaviours or indeed to ends of any kind other than that of representing the form of knowledge in the curriculum. This is because a form of knowledge has structure, and it involves procedures, concepts and criteria. Content can be selected to exemplify the most important procedures, the key concepts and the areas and situations in which the criteria hold. (p. 85)

This approach, focusing as it does on procedures, concepts and criteria, is referred to by Stenhouse as the process model. This is because it is concerned with the value of the process of learning and the learning experience itself rather than with a specific achievement outcome. It is also concerned with the intrinsic value of knowledge rather than simply its extrinsic worth.

The process model is concerned with the principles of procedure in the study of disciplines or fields of knowledge and in the analysis of social situations or controversial issues. It therefore concentrates on teacher activity, teacher-learner interaction and subject matter rather than on specified objectives. Implicit in the model is teaching by discovery or enquiry methods rather than by instruction, and it requires that the teacher become almost a senior learner.

One of the main difficulties with the process model is in relation to assessment, as Stenhouse (1975) states:

> The process model is essentially a critical model, not a marking model. It can never be directed towards an examination as an objective without loss of quality, since the standards of the examination then override the standards immanent in the subject (p. 95).

21

He then goes on to stress that this does not mean students cannot be assessed but that assessment must almost be a part of the learning process. Whereas examinations would be inappropriate, assignments, project work or discussion would be appropriate. When discussing the value of the process model he suggests:

> It may be that process models are of great importance in areas of the curriculum where understanding and criteria are central, precisely because such models counteract the pressure of the examination as an objective and deny that knowledge can be defined by the curriculum (p. 96).

It is understanding rather than overt behavioural responses that is the central point of the process model.

Arthurs (1983) has looked at the potential for using a process model to organise some aspects of a nursing curriculum. She draws attention to the three stages in the curriculum process necessary when using such a model. The first stage is to draw out a concept map of the topic. This is essentially a brainstorming exercise which may be undertaken individually or with colleagues or students. The initial topic heading is presented, and the key elements of the topic are identified and then become the basis for the content of the session or sessions. The second stage is to review the key elements and consider the principles of procedure inherent within them. The principles of procedure are concerned with how the teacher and learner will explore the subject, and may be presented in linear form from a starting point such as ascertaining what the student already knows to a concluding point which may be opportunities for experimentation or practice. The final stage is to devise an acceptable method of evaluating if teaching has been effective and learning has taken place.

Arthurs (1983) goes on to give two detailed examples of how the process model may be used in practice. Her first example, 'Taking a nursing history', is focused on the ward setting; the second example, 'Therapeutic abortion', is presented for use in the classroom. The latter provides a clear summary of the stages in the curriculum process and is reproduced in Figure 1.6.

The process model does undoubtedly have some advantage, in that it is a more dynamic and responsive approach to planning. However, to organise a total curriculum using the process approach may be very complex. The drawing up of concept maps is a lengthy business and in itself leads to a lot of discussion. It may be difficult

Figure 1.6: Application of the process model — therapeutic abortion

A: *Step One, The Concept Map*

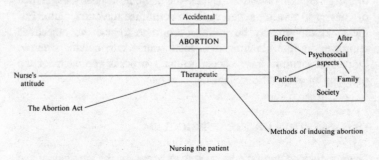

B: *Principles of Procedure for Exploring the Topic of Therapeutic Abortion (to be taught in the Classroom)*

Principles of procedure	Some suggested teaching strategies
1. Give the students relevant information about the Abortion Act 1967; methods by which abortions are induced; nursing the patient.	Formal classroom approach exercise; students to devise nursing care plan from specimen nursing history.
2. Ensure that the nurses have balanced information and the arguments for and against abortion.	Use of visual material, e.g. video, films. Guest speakers. Nurses to prepare a display within the school.
3. Encourage the nurses to begin to develop their own value stances.	Informal contact with individual students during the above activities.
4. Allow the students to 'try out' these opinions in a safe environment before meeting the problem in real life.	Classroom discussion guided by the teacher, and possibly guests. 'Forum' type session with a panel of guests.

C: *Suggestions for Evaluation Session for a Group of 7 to 10 Nurses Following Learning About Therapeutic Abortion*
Ask each nurse in turn to complete the following sentences. She may say 'pass' instead, if she wishes. Avoid discussion until all the nurses have participated.
'I felt uncomfortable when . . .'
'The most helpful part of the session was . . .'
After discussion of the above, the following questions might prove useful:
1. Have your opinions changed towards the topic? If so, how?
2. How do you expect to feel when nursing patients undergoing therapeutic abortion?
3. How do you think you would react if a junior nurse came to you who was worried about learning this topic?

Source: Arthurs (1983).

to achieve consensus on the aspects to be covered when there are lecturers from different disciplines involved in the debate. As there is no requirement to specify what students will have learnt at the end of the given experience, it may also be difficult to justify the choice of content to outsiders who come to scrutinise the curriculum. For these reasons it may be more appropriate to use the objectives approach for the planning of a total course curriculum, whereas individual lecturers may choose to use a process approach for the planning of a specific syllabus.

ORGANISATION OF THE CURRICULUM

Having decided upon the broad subject areas for the curriculum and the content to be subsumed within the subjects, the next stage in curriculum planning is to organise the content in a coherent, meaningful way. It is generally considered that there are three major criteria to be met in building an effectively organised group of learning experiences: continuity, sequence and organisation (Tyler, 1949; Taba, 1962; Pring, 1970; Hirst, 1974; Kelly, 1982). Continuity and sequence may be taken together as they are closely interlinked (Wu, 1979). When discussing ways of structuring a course, Rowntree (1981) looked at a number of potential ways of sequencing content. These may be summarised as:

(a) *Topic by topic* — a topic-based curriculum often has a very loose sequence, topics stand in their own right and the sequence is flexible.

(b) *Chronological sequence* — happenings, events, discoveries, etc. are represented in the order in which they occur, e.g. human growth and development, birth *to* death.

(c) *Causal sequence* — learning follows a chain of causation from an event or phenomenon so that when the student reaches the end of the chain he or she can explain the final effect, the event or the phenomenon itself.

(d) *Structural logic* — one aspect of a subject dependent on prior understanding of another aspect. This may also be referred to as a concept-related sequence. Posner and Strike (1976) say of this type of sequence:

. . . concept-related sequences reflect the organisation of the conceptual world. That is a sequence in which content [here, concepts] is structured in a manner consistent with the way the concepts relate to one another . . . Often referred to as the 'logical structure' this type focusses on the properties of knowledge in its final form when relationships between premises and conclusions can be analysed. (p. 673)

(e) *Problem-centred sequence* — an exploration of an issue or problem can facilitate learning, as Rowntree (1981) says:

A problem can be represented to students, or allowed to arise from their own experience and attempts to pursue solutions or interpretations of it provide a realistic context in which the teacher can help students learn the essential substance and intellectual skills of the subject. (p. 112)

(f) *Spiral sequence* — a given concept is met again and again during a course, each time at a more demanding and complex level.

(g) *Backward chaining* — the final step in a chain of events is presented first. The students then work backwards through the chain to discover the cause. This means the student completes the sequence several times rather than once only. It is thus held to be more effective that a causal sequence which involves forward chaining.

Each method of sequencing has its own advantages and disadvantages, and it may be that some aspects of the curriculum lend themselves more readily to certain types of sequence. Topic-by-topic sequencing can be advantageous if it is used to facilitate integration. This may be achieved if a specific topic is taken as the focus by each discipline at a given point in time. For example, the topic 'handicap' lends itself readily as a focus for the nursing, physiology, psychology, sociology and social-policy strands within a curriculum. It may, however, create some difficulties as it means the disciplines may be presented in a rather fragmented way. It may also be repetitive, as key concepts from the disciplines will be relevant to a number of topics.

Chronological sequencing is appropriate for some of the disciplines relevant to nursing, for example developmental psychology and social policy, but it may be an unrealistic approach for other subject areas such as physiology.

A sequence based on cause and effect is most useful in the sciences where there is opportunity for experimentation. This is particularly true of backward chaining, as the student carries out the experiment a number of times thus facilitating learning. The social sciences may also be approached in this way, particularly sociology, but it is more difficult as there is limited opportunity for direct experimentation.

The use of structural logic is particularly helpful if a basic knowledge and understanding of a discipline are required. It is the most usual form for the presentation of the academic disciplines and helps students develop their capacity for critical thinking. It has a long-term value in that studying a discipline in this way provides a firm foundation on which to build. As many nurses go on to further study after qualification, it is an asset if they have been given such an introduction to the disciplines.

The problem-centred sequence is of great in developing the student's ability to use knowledge from a variety of subject areas in a practical way. In regard to nurse training it is particularly useful way of sequencing the content of the nursing syllabus. It may be linked to the use of a nursing model or the nursing process as the tool for analysing and resolving the nursing problem.

The spiral sequence is a useful approach where in-depth knowledge of a specific discipline is required. It is probably most useful for a discipline-based degree where there is time to meet and re-meet given concepts. In regard to nursing it has limited value, as nursing draws on a range of disciplines and time would not allow for spiral sequencing in relation to these.

In essence, then, sequencing can be said to be concerned with the vertical relationship between the material presented within a given subject, whereas integration may be said to be concerned with the horizontal relationship between the different subject areas of the curriculum.

The problems of integration are many, and course planning teams need to give consideration to the different ways integration may be achieved and to acknowledge the difficulties it may create. Hirst (1974), when discussing the need for integration, gives a critical examination of the way knowledge has been divided into distinct areas. He states: '. . . all knowledge involves the use of conceptual schemes and related judgements of truth, and for that reason different forms of knowledge can be distinguished according to the character of the conceptual schemes and truth criteria involved

(p. 135)'. Similarly, Pring (1970) says of academic disciplines:

> The disciplines represent the worked out structures of knowledge, the systematic organisation of experience, the particular conceptual schemes which determine how one classifies, individuates, and proceeds with yet further enquiry. The disciplines therefore constitute in the most complete and developed form the logical structure of knowledge. (in Open University 1971, p. 269).

This division of disciplines is very important from the point of view of nursing curricula as they draw on many different disciplines, and students are required to cope with the very different conceptual frameworks and methods of enquiry of the physical and social sciences. It is therefore essential that there be some means of achieving a degree of integration in the curriculum. The Open University (1976) looks at various ways of achieving integration. These include:

> Integration in the correlation of distinct subject matter — this is essentially concerned with establishing cross-links between different subject matters. It requires collaborative planning, careful selection of examination schedules and faculty organisation.
>
> Integration through themes, topics or ideas — topics are explored in an interdisciplinary manner and in the exploration disciplinary differences become blurred and possibly unrecognisable. This requires a contribution from the whole curriculum, a range and balance of themes and subjects, a variety of teaching methods, including team teaching and a coherence of development.
>
> Integration in practical thinking may come about as the result of the resolution of difficulties which the learner identifies and enquires into. This acknowledges that there are areas of practical thinking which do not fit into well defined subject matters.
>
> Integration in the learner's own interested enquiry, this approach suggests that there are powers of mind, habits of thinking and skills of enquiry which are common to all intellectual pursuits. The key element for integration is the personal enquiry of the learner. (OU, 1976, pp. 42–57)

27

Figure 1.7: Integration and co-ordination

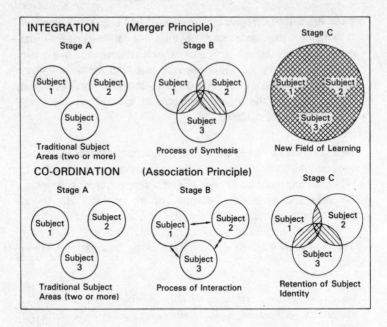

Source: Heathcote *et al.* (1982, p. 33).

Another perspective on integration is that given by Heathcote, Kempa and Roberts, (1982). They differentiate between integration and co-ordination of subject matter. Integration is defined as: '. . . the process of merging different subjects or parts of subjects through their co-ordinated use so that the individual components lose their original subject identity and a new curriculum study area emerges' (p. 32); and co-ordination as: '. . . the process of linking different subjects or part-subjects in a curriculum structure so as to effect complementary interaction between them, but retaining the characteristics of each constituent in a (to a learner) discernible way' (p. 33). This process of integration and co-ordination is presented in Figure 1.7.

The question of integration of subjects to form a new field of learning is of significance in relation to the development of nursing as a new discipline of knowledge. Smith (1983) analyses the extent to which nursing may be seen to be an 'embryonic discipline' of knowledge using King and Brownell's (1966) concept of a discipline, and concludes: 'Taken as a whole, nursing does not meet every criteria delineated by King and Brownell. Nonetheless, it is argued that nursing meets a number of criteria totally and others in part' (p. 67).

If nursing is accepted as a developing discipline, then full integration of knowledge from different subject areas becomes essential for the generation of nursing knowledge. The use of nursing theories and nursing models may provide the framework for such integration.

CURRICULUM EVALUATION

In its most basic form, evaluation could be said to be concerned with determining or appraising the value of something. As Anderson and Ball (1978) point out: 'Most people outside the field of program evaluation, including those responsible for many of the educational and social programs that are evaluated, assume that evaluation has but one purpose: to determine whether a program is any good' (p. 3). However, for people within the field of evaluation the question of appraising the value of a programme is far more complex than simply determining whether it is any good.

Early evaluators focused their work around the goals of a programme. Evaluation was to a large extent seen as the setting up of experimental tests to determine if those goals were achieved. This view of evaluation was linked very closely to the overall concept of scientific research prevalent at the time. It involved pre-input and post-input experimental tests and the use of control groups. The data collected were then quantified and often presented in statistical format.

The problem with this method of study was that often it was little more than a measurement of student ability, if that. It took no account of external factors such as previous experience of students, school environment or teaching styles. Thus if a programme was found to be ineffective, the data gave no indication of why this might be so or how the programme could be changed to make it more effective. Many people considered that this meant that evaluation itself was of limited value.

This leads on to the question of the purpose of evaluation. Scriven (1967) drew a distinction between formative and summative evaluation, the former being concerned with guiding the development of a new programme and the latter with the analysis of an established programme. Eraut, Graud and Smith (1975) suggest that if this distinction is used there are three possible roles for curriculum analysis, each serving a different audience:

> In *formative evaluation*, the audience is the development team and the purpose is to guide further development work. In the *initial stages of summative evaluation* its purpose is to guide the subsequent stages of the evaluation, so the audience is the evaluator himself. Whereas in the *final stages of summative evaluation* the audience is the decision-maker and the purpose is to guide their decisions. (p. 13)

If, then, evaluation is viewed as having a role to play in guiding decision makers, it must go beyond simply determining whether or not a programme is effective. There must be an attempt to discover what factors have contributed to making it effective or non-effective. These factors may be related to the students, the educational environment, staff–student interaction, teaching styles or the overall design of the course (Davis, 1980). They may also be related to the side-effects of the course, which may be much more significant than its intended effects (Scriven, 1973).

This requires a more flexible, responsive and naturalistic approach to evaluation. Such an approach emphasises the need to take account of the views of all those involved with the educational programme, staff, students, administrators and employers, in order to establish the issues of concern for each group. When taking account of the views of all concerned, there must be recognition of the fact that people will have differing expectations of an educational programme: 'Different people in different contexts have different standards and different values and these need to be respected by the evaluator' (p. 13).

Stake (1975) referred to the people who had a vested interest in the educational programme as the 'stakeholding audiences'. He stressed that for evaluation to be worth while it needed to focus on their different standards and values. He refers to this approach as responsive evaluation and says:

> An educational evaluation is *responsive evaluation* if it orients more directly to program activities than to program intents; responds to audience requirements for information; and if the different value perspectives present are referred to in reporting

the success and failure of the program. (p. 14)

The orientation towards programme activities is important because the evaluator needs to discover, through observation and interview with those concerned, what the programme is like in reality. Parlett and Hamilton (1972) refer to this approach as 'illuminative evaluation'. Its aims are, in their view:

. . . to study the innovatory programme; how it operates; how it is influenced by the various school situations in which it is applied; what those directly concerned regard as its advantages and disadvantages; and how students' intellectual tasks and academic experiences are most affected.

Another significant feature of the responsive/illuminative approach to evaluation is that it allows for a variety of ways of feeding back information to interested parties (Stake, 1975). If evaluation of an educational programme is to be worth while, then it is essential that there is effective communication of the results. With responsive evaluation this feedback may be in verbal or written form. Reports can be presented in a way that communicates more naturally than traditional research reports, which are often complex and difficult to understand unless one is familiar with the research method used.

As Guba and Lincoln (1981) point out, responsive evaluation has many advantages over more traditional methods. Because it is concerned with presenting an overall picture of an educational programme, it allows for the incorporation of other approaches when appropriate. For example, some evaluators (Tyler, 1949; Stake, 1967) have used objectives as a focus for the evaluation. Others (Cronbach, 1963; Stufflebeam, 1971, cited in Stenhouse, 1975) have used decisions and been concerned with how evaluation can serve the decision makers. With responsive evaluation both these aspects can be given attention. Therefore, as Guba and Lincoln (1981) say: 'The resulting flexibility gives the responsive model power beyond that of any of its competitors' (p. 38).

Gallego (1983) in her evaluation of a school of nursing elected to use an 'ideological model of evaluation' because such a model is: '. . . concerned with exploring the ethos, the "institutional personality", the ideologies which form a part of any institution' (p. 43). In that such an approach takes account of the views of students, teachers and other relevant parties and focuses on the teaching/learning process, not simply learning outcomes, it is closely aligned to the responsive model. This approach is discussed in more detail by Amalia Gallego in Chapter 10.

CONCLUSION

This chapter was not intended to be a definitive statement on the process of curriculum planning. It is probable that it has raised more questions than it has answered but reference has been made to a range of sources of further information which will give a more in-depth discussion of the important issues.

An attempt has been made to consider key areas in the planning process. The curriculum models, while they should not be seen as the only way of approaching curriculum planning, do nevertheless provide a useful tool for identifying areas of discussion for a course planning team. It is also important that those involved in nurse education debate the nature of nursing and the use of nursing models and nursing theories in relation to the organisation of the curriculum. A course planning team needs to have a clear picture of the end product of the course to guide the selection of content and the organisation of learning experiences. The value of the process approach to curriculum planning is recognised, but it is also acknowledged that it is probably simpler to design the total curriculum using an objectives approach. Such an approach is more readily open to scrutiny by others and may be justified more easily. The issues of sequencing and integration are fundamental to the planning process. It is only through effective sequencing and integration that a coherent programme, which will facilitate student learning, can be designed. Finally, evaluation is an essential component of the planning process. It is not the end of the curriculum process but in many ways the beginning.

As yet there are relatively few key texts on the process of curriculum planning is nursing, though the body of literature is growing (Bevis, 1982; Heath, 1982; Torres and Stanton, 1982; Davis, 1983; Greaves, 1984; Scales, 1985; Jolley and Allan, 1986). An increasing number of nurse educationalists (see Davis, 1986, for a review of the literature on nursing education) are focusing on issues central to the planning process, such as the use of nursing theories and nursing models as a basis for curriculum planning, the nature of nursing knowledge and the need for a more integrated approach to curriculum. The dissemination of their ideas through journal articles and conference papers is essential to promote healthy debate among all involved in the field of nurse education if nursing curricula are to respond to the challenge of Project 2000 (UKCC, 1986).

NOTE

1. Per Dalin (1974) used the theoretical framework provided by Bennis *et al.* (1969) for a major international study on educational innovation carried out between 1970 and 1973. For a fuller discussion of these strategies see Dalin (1982).

REFERENCES

Anderson, S.B. and Ball, S. (1983) *The profession and practice of program evaluation*. Jossey-Bass, London

Arthurs, J. (1983) The process model — an alternative approach to the curriculum. *Nurse Education Today, 3* (4), 77–80

Arthurs, J. (1984) The nursing model — a tool for nurse educators. *Nurse Education Today, 4* (3), 58–9

Barnett, R., Becher, A.R. and Cork, N.M. (1986) Models of professional preparation, unpublished research report for the Department of Education and Science

Bennis, W.G., Benne, K.D. and Chinn, R. (eds) (1969) *The planning of change*. Holt, Rinehart & Winston, New York

Bevis, E.O. (1982) *Curriculum building in nursing — a process*. C.V. Mosby, St. Louis, MO

Birchenall, P.D. (1985) Applying aspects of curriculum studies to the practice of nurse teaching. *Nurse Education Today, 5*, 147–50

Bloom, B.S. (ed.) (1956) *Taxonomy of educational objectives: The classification of educational goals. Handbook I: cognitive domain.* McKay, New York

Briggs, A. (1972) *Report of the Committee on Nursing*, Cmnd 5115. HMSO, London

Brown, S.T. and Lee, B.T. (1980) Imogene King's conceptual framework: a proposed model for continuing nurse education. *Journal of Advanced Nursing, 5*, 467–73

Chapman, P. (1984) Specifics and generalities: a critical examination of two nursing models. *Nurse Education Today, 4* (6), 141–4

Collister, B. (1983) From one speculator to another: the framework of nursing curricula. *Nurse Education Today, 3* (2), 32–7

Commission on Nursing Education (1985) *The education of nurses: a new dispensation*. Royal College of Nursing, London

Cork, N.M. (1986) Models of professional preparation: a profile of graduate nurse education, unpublished research report for the Department of Education and Science

Cronbach, L. (1963) Course improvement through evaluation. *Teachers' College Research*, 64, 672–83

Dalin, P. (1982) Strategies of innovation, in Horton, T. and Raggatt, P. (eds) *Challenge and change in the curriculum*. Hodder & Stoughton, London

Davies, I.K. (1976) *Objectives in curriculum design*. McGraw-Hill, New York and London

Davis, B.D. (ed.) (1983) *Research into nurse education*. Croom Helm, London

Davis, B.D. (1986) Nursing education, *British Book News*, May 1986, 275–8

Davis, E.D. (1980) *Teachers as curriculum evaluators*. Allen & Unwin, London and Sydney

DHSS (1986a) *Neighbourhood nursing: a focus for care: Report of the Community Nursing Review*. HMSO, London

DHSS (1986b) *Primary health care: an agenda for discussion*. HMSO, London

Dufton, A. (1985) From hospital to college. *NATFE Journal*, No. 7, 22–3

English National Board for Nursing, Midwifery and Health Visiting (1985) Professional education training courses, consultation paper

Eraut, M.R. (1976) Some perspectives on curriculum development in teacher education. *Education for Teaching*, No. 99, 19

Eraut, M.R., Goad, L. and Smith, G. (1975) The analysis of curriculum materials. University of Sussex, Education Area, Occasional Paper No. 2

Evans, L.R. (1982) Factors exerting influence on the development of nursing curriculum. *Nurse Education Today*, 2 (3), 21–4

Gallego, A.P. (1983) *Evaluating the school: a case study in the evaluation of a school of nursing*. Royal College of Nursing, London

Gott, M. (1982) Theories of learning and the teaching of nursing. *Nursing Times*, 78 (11), 41–4

Greaves, F. (1984) *Nurse education and the curriculum: a curricular model*. Croom Helm, London

Guba, E.G. and Lincoln, Y.S. (1981) *Effective evaluation*. Jossey-Bass, London

Harrow, A. (1972) *A taxonomy of the psychomotor domain*. McKay, New York

Havelock, R.G. (1973) *The change agent's guide to innovation*. Educational Technology Publications, New Jersey

Heath, J. (1982) Intention and practice in nursing education. *Nurse Education Today*, 2 (4), 7–9

Heathcote, G., Kempa, R. and Roberts, I. (1982) *Curriculum styles and strategies*. Ch. 4: The organisation of curriculum content. Further Education Curriculum Review and Development Group, London

Henderson, V. (1978) The concept of nursing. *Journal of Advanced Nursing*, 3, 113–30

Hirst, P.H. (1974) *Knowledge and the curriculum*. Routledge & Kegan Paul, London

Hoy, R.A. and Mustafa, A. (1983) Curriculum theory in nurse education. *Nurse Education Today*, 3 (2), 37

Hoyle, E. (1972) *Problems of curriculum innovation*. Open University Press, Milton Keynes

Johnston, C.M. (1978) Total patient care v. task allocation: a student nurse's point of view, in Allen, H.O. and Murrell, J. (eds) *Nursing training: an enterprise in curriculum development*. Macdonald & Evans, Plymouth

Jolley, M. and Allan, P. (1986) *Curriculum issues in nursing education*. Croom Helm, London

Kelly, A.V. (1982) *The curriculum: theory and practice*. Harper & Row, London

Kerr, J.F. (ed.) (1968) *Changing the curriculum*. University of London Press, London

King, A.R. and Brownell, J.A. (1968) *The curriculum and the disciplines of knowledge*. Wiley, New York cited in L. Smith (1983) Nursing: an embryonic discipline of knowledge. *Nursing Education Today, 3* (3), 67–7

King, I.M. (1971) *Towards a theory of nursing*. Wiley, New York

Knowles, M.S. (1970) *The modern practice of adult education: androgogy versus pedagogy*. Association Press, New York

Krathwohl, D.R., Bloom, B.S. and Masia, B.B. (1964) *Taxonomy of educational objectives: The classification of educational goals — handbook II: affective domain*. McKay, New York

Kratz, C.R. (ed.) (1979) *The nursing process*. Bailliere Tindall, London

Lee, V. and Zeldin, D. (1982) *Planning in the curriculum*. Hodder & Stoughton, London

Little, D.E. and Carnevali, D.L. (1976) *Nursing care planning*, Lippincott, Philadelphia, PA

McFarlane, E. (1980) Nursing theory: the comparison of four theoretical proposals. *Journal of Advanced Nursing, 5*, 3–19

McGlynn, J. (1984) The quest for nursing knowledge. *Nurse Education Today, 4* (2), 46–7

Meleis, A.I. (1979) The development of a conceptually based nursing curriculum: an international experiment. *Journal of Advanced Nursing, 4*, 659–71

Mezirow, J. (1983) A critical theory of adult learning and education. In Tight, M. (ed.) *Adult learning and education*. Croom Helm, London

Open University (1971) *The curriculum: context, design and development*. Open University Press, Milton Keynes

Open University (1976) *Educational studies: a second level course. Curriculum design and development, units 11–13*. Open University Press, Milton Keynes

Orem, D.E. (1980) *Nursing concepts of practice*. McGraw-Hill, New York

Parlett, M. and Hamilton, D. (1972) Evaluation as illumination: a new approach to the study of innovatory programmes. Occasional paper of the centre for research in the educational sciences, University of Edinburgh

Paterson, R.W.K. (1979) *Values, education and the adult*. Routledge & Kegan Paul, London

Peters, R.S. (1966) *Ethics and education*. Allen & Unwin, London

Peters, R.S. (1967) *The concept of education*. Routledge & Kegan Paul, London

Peters, R.S. (1977) *Education and the education of teachers*. Routledge & Kegan Paul, London

Popham, W.J. (1968) Probing the validating of the arguments against behavioural objectives. A symposium presentation at the Annual American Educational Research Association Meeting, Chicago, 7–10 February 1968, cited in I.K. Davies (1976) *Objectives in curriculum design*. McGraw-Hill, New York and London

Posner, G.J. and Strike, K.A. (1976) A categorisation scheme for principles of sequencing content. *Review of Educational Research, 46* (4)

Pratt, D. (1980) *Curriculum design and development*. Harcourt Brace Jovanovich, New York

Pring, R. (1970) Curriculum integration. London Institute of Education Bulletin, Spring, cited in Open University (1971) *The Curriculum: context, design and development*, Open University, Milton Keynes

Quinn, F.M. (1980) *The principles and practice of nurse education*. Croom Helm, London

Redman, B.K. (1984) *The process of patient education*. C.V. Mosby, St. Louis, MO

Riehl, J.P. and Roy, C. (eds) (1980) *Conceptual models for nursing practice*. Appleton Century Crofts, New York

Roberts, K.L. (1985) Theory of nursing as curriculum content. *Journal of Advanced Nursing, 10*, 209–15

Rogers, M.E. (1970) *An introduction to a theoretical basis of nursing*. F.A. Davis, Philadelphia, PA

Roper, N., Logan, W. and Tierney, A.J. (1983) *Using a model for nursing*. Churchill Livingstone, London

Rowntree, D. (1981) *Developing courses for students*, McGraw-Hill, New York

Roy, S.C. (1976) *Introduction to nursing: an adaptation model*. Prentice-Hall, Englewood Cliffs, NJ

Scales, F.S. (1985) *Nursing curriculum: development, structure, function*, Appleton-Century Crofts, New York/Prentice-Hall, Englewood Cliffs, NJ

Scriven, M. (1967) *The methodology of evaluation*. AERA Monograph Series in Curriculum Evaluation No. 1, Rand McNally, Chicago, Ill.

Scriven, M. (1973) Goal-free evaluation, in House, E.R. (ed.) *School evaluation: the politics and process*. McCutchan, Berkeley, CA

Sheahan, J. (1978) Educating teachers of nursing: the contribution of pedagogical studies. *Journal of Advanced Nursing, 3*, 515–24

Sheahan, J. (1980) Some aspects of the teaching and learning of nursing. *Journal of Advanced Nursing, 5*, 491–511

Simpson, E. (1972) The classification of educational objectives in the psychomotor domain. *The psychomotor domain*, vol. 3, Cryphon House, Washington, DC, cited in Quinn, F.M. (1980) *The principles and practice of nurse education*. Croom Helm, London

Smith, L. (1982) Models of nursing as the basis for curriculum development: some rationales and implications. *Journal of Advanced Nursing, 7*, 117–27

Smith, L. (1983) Nursing: an embryonic discipline of knowledge. *Nurse Education Today, 3* (3), 62–7

Stake, R.E. (1967) The countenance of educational evaluation. *Teachers College Record, 68*, 523–40, cited in Davis, E. (1980) *Teachers as curriculum evaluators*. Allen & Unwin, Sydney

Stake, R.E. (ed.) (1975) *Evaluating the arts in education: a responsive approach*. Merrill, Columbus, Ohio

Stenhouse, L. (1975) *An introduction to curriculum research and development*. Heinemann, London

Stevens, B.J. (1979) *Nursing theory: analysis, application, evaluation*. Little Brown, Boston

Stufflebeam, D.L. (Ed.) (1971) Educational evaluation and decision making. F.E. Peacock for Phi Delta Kappa National Study Committee on Evaluation, Itasca, Ill, cited in Stenhouse, L. (1975) *An introduction to curriculum research and development*. Heinemann, London

Taba, H. (1962) *Curriculum developments: theory and practice*. Harcourt Brace and World, New York

Torres, G. and Stanton, M. (1982) *Curriculum process in nursing*. Prentice-Hall, Englewood Cliffs, NJ

Tyler, R.W. (1949) *Basic principles of curriculum instruction*. University of Chicago Press, Chicago

United Kingdom Central Council for Nursing, Midwifery and Health Visiting (1986) *Project 2000: a new preparation for practice*. UKCC, London, May 1986

Wu, R.R. (1979) Designing a curriculum model. *Journal of Nursing Education, 18*, 13–21

2

The Life Sciences in Nurse Education

J.A. Akinsanya

INTRODUCTION

A review of the literature on nursing research in the UK reveals a considerable number of studies based on a behavioural sciences foundation (Inman, 1975; Macleod Clark and Hockey, 1979; Hayward and Lelean, 1982; Davis, 1983a, b). However, there is a dearth of research into the role of the life sciences in nursing education in the UK. Two important studies in this field are those by Nolan (1973) and Wilson (1975). Wilson's study suggests that the life sciences theory that underpins nursing practice is unstructured and ill-defined. This lack of definition in the syllabus for general and specialised nursing courses has been noted by nurse educators who have increasingly expressed concern about it (Cox, 1982a, b). A particularly important aspect of Wilson's study is the evidence that the application of theoretical knowledge of the life sciences is 'unstructured and appears to be haphazard'.

The study reported in this chapter started from a consideration of the need to develop a life sciences nursing model as a basis for the nursing curriculum, and, more specifically, from a concern within that context for strengthening the life sciences base in nursing curricula. The term 'bionursing' was coined to describe what is considered to be a distinctive life sciences knowledge base and its application in nursing practice which reflects the nursing model of patient care. It is argued that the application of biological principles to other disciplines acknowledges this by a prefix 'bio', as is the case in medicine where a 'biomedical' term refers specifically to the uses of biological principles in medical education.

Within this context, the study attempts to identify a 'bionursing' approach to the life sciences curriculum in nurse education, and to explore the perceptions of learners, nurse tutor students and directors of nurse tutor courses with regard to:

(1) the role of the life sciences in the performance of nursing tasks;
(2) their preparation for performing, and for teaching about, nursing care as related to the life sciences and their application to its practice;
(3) the usefulness of a 'bionursing' model in nurse education.

A theoretical framework developed for the study will now be considered, followed by a summary of the empirical studies.

THEORETICAL FRAMEWORK FOR THE EMPIRICAL STUDY

The problem with which this study is concerned can be illustrated by an example from the Preliminary Examination Paper of the General Nursing Council for England and Wales (GNC) for the General Register in 1942. One of the questions asked candidates to: 'Describe the physiology of respiration.' This question illustrates the importance attached to a knowledge of physiology by the examiners of the time. A number of authors at the time also emphasised the importance of the contribution of life sciences to the practice of nursing. One such writer, Hainsworth (1936), noted that 'a sound knowledge of nursing science and practice' depends on the underlying sciences such as anatomy and physiology.

Four decades on, there are those who question the need for an in-depth knowledge of the life sciences in nursing. Thus Holford (1981), in a discussion of the place of the life sciences in nursing, argues:

It matters very little whether or not the nurse understands the physiology of the [chloride shift] to care for the patient in respiratory distress. What are necessary are basic common sense and the ability to soothe and reassure. It is for the doctors to provide the rest.

In a similar vein, another contributor to the debate, Phillipson (1982), noted: 'To care for the hospital patient, a handful of simple skills supported by a little knowledge is all that is necessary. Nursing auxiliaries demonstrate this daily in the NHS.'

More recently, in the United States, Starck (1984) questioned the current teaching of the life sciences in nursing curricula. She noted the economic consequences of attempts to teach these sciences within the school of nursing as distinct disciplines and urged that more resources should be concentrated on the teaching of nursing itself.

These sciences (anatomy, physiology, microbiology and pharmacology) represent one of the key areas of scientific underpinning of nursing practice. For if nursing tasks are to be performed with the understanding that will ensure scrupulous attention to detail in the interests of patients' safety and well-being, then the information base that supplies the reasons for every action in the performance of a nursing task must be clearly understood by the nurse. This information base has, as a substantial component, the life sciences of anatomy and physiology (the body and how it works), microbiology (the effect on the body of micro-organisms) and pharmacology (the response of the body to the introduction of pharmacological agents) (GNC, 1977).

The study of the life sciences has been a feature of the nurse education curriculum since the subjects were introduced into the GNC Syllabus of 1922 (Bendall and Raybould, 1969). However, very little research appears to have been carried out in relation to the way these subjects are taught and learnt in nursing. There are a number of possible explanations for this apparent lack of research in the area of teaching and learning the life sciences in nursing. Two of these may be considered here.

The first is that nursing traditionally relied on medicine for its life sciences curricular needs, and medical staff were closely involved in the education of nurse learners for many years (Adams and Taylor, 1974). It may be that one result was a version of these subjects based on the medical curriculum, while the teaching of the application of the life sciences to nursing practice was for the most part based on their pathophysiological implications (McCarthy, 1972).

Secondly, it could be argued that, because nursing has derived its knowledge of these sciences second-hand through medicine, teachers and practitioners have not been encouraged to search for a distinctive link between nursing and these subjects in the curriculum. Yet such a link may be necessary because of the differences in medical and nursing curricula and the way these sciences are taught in the two related disciplines (Holmes, 1972).

Moreover, growing concern for professionalisation of nursing has placed an emphasis on professional competence, which recognises that responsible, accountable, nursing care is not merely an affair of carrying out instructions and performing routine tasks; but that it also requires informed observation, accurate reporting of information, and informed communication with patients and others (McFarlane, 1977; Faulkner, 1980). Above all, it could be argued that professional competence should reflect informed decision-making at all times in circumstances which may be either routine or emergency in nature. This implies the need for a measure of flexibility within a framework of procedures. This constitutes what Bosanquet and Clifton (1973) described as 'the discretionary element' in nursing care. The authors observed nursing activities in the wards over a long period and noted the following examples as requiring informed decision-making on the part of the nurses concerned:

(a) How best to turn an unconscious patient?
(b) Is Mr X (a recent coronary) changing colour, and if so should the doctor be called?
(c) How does the nurse get a Ryles' tube down a confused old man who is coughing hard?
(d) Why has the registrar ordered 5 mg of diamorphine as a pre-medication for a patient with chronic bronchitis who is to have a supra-pubic catheter removed? Is it sensible to give this patient a drug which depresses breathing?

The authors stressed the importance of a knowledge base for informed practice and reported: 'One student nurse after eight weeks on a medical ward with numbers of patients with strokes did not know the causes of them.'

The evidence above would seem to suggest that nurse education and training should be geared to the development of professional responsibility and accountability and of confidence of the individual's professional ability to act as an acknowledged 'expert' on nursing care. Fundamental to this concept of professional competence is the need to ensure that nursing education emphasises the underlying reasons for nursing tasks and other activities which have to do with patient care, i.e. the need for a model of nursing education that is distinct from the medical model that has dominated the nursing curriculum for a long time. This would constitute a positive attempt to counterbalance what McCarthy (1972) called the 'over-reliance on the medical profession for the teaching of nurses' and a system which he described as 'ineffective, inefficient and, in some ways, harmful to the progress of nursing'. This view, from a surgeon interested in the education of nurses, deserves serious consideration in any discussion of the role of the life sciences in nursing education. For what he and many others have argued is that the model for nurse education should be one based on 'care', and that much of the teaching should be in the hands of nurses with this orientation (see below).

A MODEL OF NURSING FOR NURSING EDUCATION

The introduction of nursing models in recent years has encouraged the replacement of much of the current medically orientated input of knowledge generally. This trend, described by Peterson (1983) as: 'General progression away from the medical systems model to a conceptual, nursing-care-process model', has characterised curriculum design in nursing education in the past decade. However, it could be argued that the effect of such changes may not lead to fundamental changes in nursing unless new approaches are adopted in relation to the teaching and learning of the behavioural and life sciences.

Figure 2.1 shows the distinguishing features of the two models in use in medical and nursing education. The medical model emphasises signs and symptoms in relation to pathology, and the nursing model summarises a problem-solving approach which is recognised as the nursing process, and which Roper, Logan and Tierney (1981) term 'the process of nursing'.

It could be argued that a nursing model based on the concept of 'care' will be centrally concerned with the tasks performed by nurses: skills and techniques, the reasons for the performance of which may lie in one or both of the life and behavioural sciences (Greaves, 1979; Roper *et al.*, 1981; Baldwin, 1983; Akinsanya, 1984).

This study focuses solely on the life sciences component, although similar considerations might apply to the behavioural sciences as well. In the area of the life sciences, this chapter argues that a 'bionursing' approach might be proposed which would be concerned with the essential aspects of patient care based on knowledge directly derived from the life sciences. This would contrast with the existing 'biomedical' approach in which the emphasis is on pathology and medical diagnosis. Such a 'bionursing' orientation might have, as a pivotal innovation, the linking of the

Figure 2.1: The distinguishing features of medical and nursing models

The nursing model

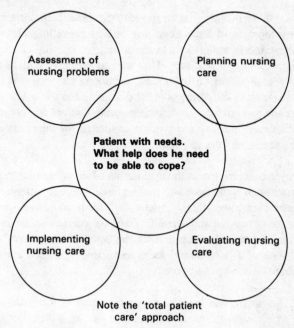

Assessment of nursing problems

Planning nursing care

Patient with needs. What help does he need to be able to cope?

Implementing nursing care

Evaluating nursing care

Note the 'total patient care' approach

The medical model

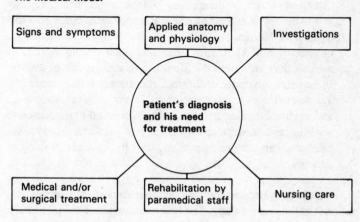

| Signs and symptoms | Applied anatomy and physiology | Investigations |

Patient's diagnosis and his need for treatment

| Medical and/or surgical treatment | Rehabilitation by paramedical staff | Nursing care |

tasks that constitute nursing care, i.e. the skills and techniques, and any situation-specific modifications, with a distinctively derived knowledge base in the life sciences. As Chinn (1983) points out:

> . . . there needs to be an increasingly clear commitment to the development of knowledge that reflects prevailing views of the discipline (nursing) and to the testing of nursing concepts and theoretical formulations. The need to conceive and implement new approaches for the testing of nursing knowledge is critical; the nature of the concepts of the discipline and the lack of existing means to verify or validate phenomena that are important to the practice of nursing are a major challenge for the community of nurse researchers (p. 402).

A major concern here is the exploration of ideas in order to provide a conceptual link between nursing and the life sciences. It is therefore suggested that a 'bionursing' focus could well provide a rational, structured and scientific basis for curriculum development in the professional education of the nurse. The acceptability or otherwise of a 'bionursing' focus in nursing education may, in the final analysis, depend upon:

(1) The nature and level of specific aspects of the basic sciences which nurse learners would need to master, with understanding, in order to perform basic and technical nursing procedures.
(2) Clinical application of life sciences concepts which underpin the theory of nursing — the mastery of these concepts and the way in which they would enable the learner to demonstrate effective transfer of learning.
(3) Organisation of knowledge of facts, principles and theories of nursing derivable from the life sciences and capable of transfer in learners, given their different educational backgrounds.
(4) The learner's ability to comprehend, apply, analyse, synthesise and evaluate nursing practice on an individual basis related to well-defined task characteristics, as defined above; for example, care of pressure areas, oral hygiene and feeding of patients.

Two theories proposed in the last two decades are particularly relevant to the present study. The first of these is that of Fitts (1965), described as a 'three-phase theory'. Fitts suggests that the performance of tasks is characterised by three phases which overlap continuously but are capable of theoretical delineation. These are defined as:

(a) The cognitive phase — involving the analysis of tasks.
(b) The associative phase — when correct patterns of response are developed through practice by the learner.
(c) The autonomous phase — when tasks are performed skilfully and automatically.

The second approach uses the technique of task analysis in terms of component skills and knowledge (Demaree, 1961; Annett, 1971; Edney, 1972). Demaree, for example, considers that skill acquisition depends on four categories of teaching/learning requirements. These are categorised as:

(1) The learning of knowledge related to the task, i.e. terms, concepts, principles and their relationships in practice.
(2) The learning skills and their related tasks in order to make decisions about appropriateness, accuracy and necessity for their performance in specific instances.
(3) The learning and mastery of whole-task performance involving procedures, contexts of performance and the complexity of decisions that have to be made.
(4) The learning and mastery of integrated-task performance when tasks have to be co-ordinated within an overall teaching approach.

This study is not concerned with the levels to which the life sciences are studied by prospective nurses, although these or equivalent levels of knowledge are held to represent important prerequisites to a career in nursing.

Within this context, the empirical studies that follow represent an attempt to determine the extent to which a life sciences basis for nursing practice and nurse education might be defined and subsequently explored. The aims of the study are as follows:

(1) to describe learners' perceptions of the role of the life sciences in their education and training for professional practice;
(2) to seek evidence for the preparation of nurse tutors in the knowledge they require in order to teach the application of the life sciences;
(3) to ascertain the perceptions of nurse tutor students and their course directors on the role and relevance of the life sciences

in nursing care and in the preparation of nurse tutors, and on the effectiveness of present courses in equipping nurse tutors for teaching the application of life sciences knowledge in nursing practice in such a way as to link theory with practice by providing an understanding of the reasons for actions;

(4) to ascertain nurses' views on whether the introduction of a bionursing conceptual framework (instead of the existing medical one) would help to provide a direct link between nursing and its life sciences foundation;

(5) to test the researcher's model of task hierarchy/life sciences input;

(6) to supplement the growing literature on the contribution of the life sciences in nursing education and the need for a clearer definition on their application to its practice;

(7) to identify and clarify issues for further research.

THE EMPIRICAL STUDY

Because of the dearth of research in this area, the research programme was necessarily evolutionary in its development. It consisted of three distinct stages. In Stage I, an exploratory study involved attempts to develop an appropriate strategy for the later empirical study. This resulted in the development of a questionnaire for learners, designed:

(1) to canvass the views of learners on their perceived usefulness of the concept of 'bionursing' for examining the input of the life sciences in nursing education and relating these to nursing practice;

(2) to explore the preceived depth and levels of knowledge of these subjects required for specific nursing activities and procedures (which might also act as a test of the hierarchy model in this study);

(3) to assess the reactions of learners at various stages of basic general training to the term 'bionursing' as a description of the application of knowledge derived from the biological/life sciences in nursing education and practice.

The sample

A total of 165 volunteer learners in two teaching and one non-teaching hospitals in south-east England participated. The evidence from this exploratory study suggested tentatively that a major root of the problem of life sciences in nursing education might lie in the way tutors and clinical teachers are prepared, and how they view their role as teachers using knowledge derived from the life sciences (something which had been mentioned by nurse tutors and clinical teachers during preliminary discussions).

It was decided to survey by means of questionnaire the opinions of nurse tutor students ($n = 324$) on the role and teaching of the application of the life sciences in the practice of nursing, their perception of their preparation for teaching in this area, as well as the difficulties and anxieties they experienced. Twelve directors of nurse tutor courses were also interviewed on the role and teaching of the application of the life sciences in nursing and the preparation of nurse tutor students; the effectiveness of the preparation at present; and future plans. Aspects of the findings are reported below.

Preliminary empirical studies were carried out as attempts to explore the various aspects of the investigation into the role of the life sciences in nursing education. The main area of interest in these preliminary explorations was the categorisation of the life sciences input in relation to nursing tasks, and the extent to which this was made clear or at least understood in each case as an important reason for the different aspects of each task performed by learners.

This study was particularly concerned with the extent to which newly recruited learners connected the life sciences being learned in the school with practice in carrying out or assisting with nursing tasks on the wards. These exploratory ward observations, discussions and consultations with trained nurses suggested that a close examination of the problem would be instructive.

Findings: the perceptions of learners

In the tape-recorded interviews with learners, it seemed that the approaches adopted were largely *biomedical*, unstructured and disappointing. This finding confirms Wilson's (1975) conclusion of the haphazardness of nurse training in the way these sciences are taught and used by learners and the qualified alike. In the light of the evidence from the literature and the exploratory study that shows that this problem exists, it was decided to widen the scope of the study to include teaching hospitals in the main study. The following research questions were therefore formulated:

(1) Which of the life sciences taught to learners do they perceive as being difficult either to learn or to apply to their practice?
(2) Which of the activities performed by nurses that involve the application of the life sciences could they initiate independently of medical prescription if they had an appropriate understanding of the underlying life sciences?
(3) Would the term 'bionursing' (developed in the theoretical framework) provide a more direct link between nursing and the life sciences than the present use of the term 'biomedical'?

Figure 2.2: Learners' indication of life sciences subjects in which they experience difficulty (*n* = 165)

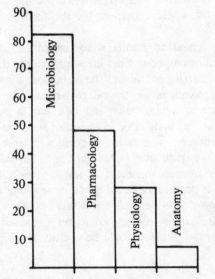

One learner may rank more than one subject

The results in Figure 2.2 indicate that less than half of the respondents perceived difficulties in the learning of the life sciences. The nature of these difficulties was not explored in this study. This would seem an area worthy of further investigation, particularly in

Table 2.1: Learners' indication of areas of nursing practice for which the nurse requires an adequate knowledge base in the life sciences[a] (n = 165)

	Ranking of nursing activities in order of level of knowledge of the life sciences required for practice							
	Anatomy		Physiology		Pharmacology		Microbiology	
	n	%	n	%	n	%	n	%
Care of the unconscious patient	115	69.7	45	27.3	1	0.6	1	0.6
Management of intravenous infusion	26	15.7	105	63.6	8	4.8	10	6.1
Administration of drugs (all routes)	2	1.2	6	3.6	148	89.7	7	4.2
Taking and recording blood pressure, pulse, respiration and temperature	4	2.4	155	93.9	4	2.4	–	–
Preparation of patients for special tests	59	35.8	61	37.0	21	12.7	9	5.5
Care of pressure areas	11	6.7	42	25.5	69	41.8	16	9.7
Feeding via nasogastric tube	140	84.8	6	3.6	12	7.3	5	3.0
Dressing wounds	2	1.2	3	1.8	8	4.8	151	91.5
Testing urine	30	18.2	55	33.3	63	38.2	5	3.0
Giving and removing bottles and bedpans	13	7.9	46	27.9	65	39.4	6	3.6
Administration of oxygen	6	3.6	136	82.4	15	9.1	7	4.2
Giving an enema	145	87.9	7	4.2	9	5.5	7	4.2
Explaining procedures to patients	104	63.0	43	26.1	1	0.6	1	0.6
Oral hygiene	20	12.1	98	59.4	–	–	9	5.5
Getting patient up	148	89.7	8	4.8	2	1.2	5	3.0

[a] Excludes the not-coded column.

microbiology which was indicated as being difficult to learn by 49.7% of the learners.

As will seen from Table 2.1, a knowledge of applied anatomy and physiology was emphasised by respondents in relation to most of the nursing activities with which they were concerned. It is not clear, however, whether an understanding of their underlying principles can be inferred from their awareness of the constant demands made upon them in clinical practice. It could in fact reflect little more than the constant emphasis upon the importance of these subjects in nurse training.

From Table 2.1, it would seem that respondents perceived the need for a high level of knowledge of the life sciences in relation to particular nursing activities. For instance, 69.7% regarded a high level of knowledge of anatomy as essential in the care of the unconscious patient; and for getting patients up, giving an enema, and nasogastric feeding, respondents saw a high level of knowledge of anatomy as being particularly essential to the nurse, i.e. 89.7%, 87.9% and 84.8% respectively for each of these nursing activities.

Although a high level of knowledge of physiology was perceived as being essential to the nurse in the taking and recording of blood pressure, temperature and pulse (93.9%), it needs to be said that a knowledge of applied anatomy and physiology is inseparable from these practical nursing activities. Not surprisingly, 89.7% of respondents rated a high level of knowledge of pharmacology as essential to the nurse in the administation of drugs. On the other hand, respondents rated the need for a high level of knowledge of microbiology as essential in the dressing of wounds (91.9%). Yet only 5.5% of the respondents regarded a similar level of knowledge of microbiology as being essential for giving mouth care to patients. Indeed, care of pressure areas was consistently rated low in terms of the level of knowledge of the life sciences required to perform it.

The learners' perceptions of knowledge of the life sciences required for the performance of various nursing activities appear to suggest that these subjects are viewed as being important in their training. In the case of anatomy, for example, the results show that activities that would involve nurses in direct physical invasion of the body would require a perceived knowledge of this life science: 84.8% of respondents rated it important for the passing of nasogastric tube, 87.9% for giving an enema, 63.0% for explaining procedures to patients, and 89.7% for getting patients up. In all these activities, the physical condition of the individual is a major concern of the nurse, and a knowledge of anatomy would be essential in order to ensure safety in their care.

In the case of physiology, learners' perceptions reflect the need for a knowledge of this life science in the nursing care of patients. For taking and recording blood pressure, temperature, pulse and respiration, 93.9% of respondents perceived a knowledge of physiology as being important. For administration of oxygen, management of intravenous infusion and giving oral care, the corresponding ratings were 82.4%, 63.6% and 59.4% respectively.

It is interesting to note the result for pharmacology as perceived by learners. Clearly, administration of drugs is fundamental here, and 89.7% rated a knowledge of this subject as being important in the performance of this nursing task. For the care of pressure areas, giving and removing bedpans and testing urine, 41.8%, 39.4% and 38.2% of learners perceived a knowledge of pharmacology as being important. These results might be explained by the fact that pharmacological agents are sometimes used in the treatment of pressure necrosis, and elimination and excretion of pharmacological end products are the concern of the digestive and excretory systems in the body.

Finally 97.6% of learners in this study not surprisingly perceived a knowledge of microbiology as being important for the dressing of wounds.

The results suggest that learners' anxieties and uncertainties in relation to the role of the life sciences in nursing and nurse education may be less a matter of basic scientific knowledge (they are generally better qualified to cope with the demands of a biologically based course in nursing) than a matter of input, both theoretical and applied, and the development of a real *understanding* of the reasons for their actions.

The life sciences and the preparation of nurse tutors

The aim of this stage of the study was to obtain the views of nurse tutor students on the role of the life sciences in nursing and in their own preparation as teachers. Specifically, the following questions were addressed:

(1) Whether the total exclusion of the life sciences as formal subjects in courses preparing nurse tutors is likely to affect their later ability to teach the subjects.

(2) Whether nurse tutor students were themselves sufficiently

51

prepared professionally before undertaking the course of preparation as future teachers of the life sciences.

Because of the timing of the study, it was decided to carry out the survey in two separate halves, i.e. one at the end of the course (May 1980) when students would have had teaching practice, and the other at the beginning of the following academic year (September 1980) before teaching practices were undertaken.

Figure 2.3 shows the breakdown of the type of course attended by respondents. The increasing number of one-year full-time courses is confirmed. Students on two-year full-time courses in this study were the last to be accepted for the University of London Sister Tutor Diploma (STD). The two-year part-time courses are in-service programmes established as part of one-year full-time courses and run by the same course directors for those students who prefer this form of longer preparation.

The perceptions of nurse tutor students of the importance of subjects taught to learners were revealing, as shown in Figures 2.4 and 2.5. When the responses are compared, an important difference

Figure 2.3: Students who completed questionnaires by the type of course attended (*n* = 324)

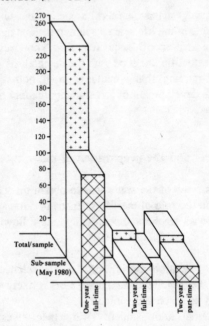

Figure 2.4: Nurse tutor students' choice of subjects in order of importance for their own preparation (*n* = 324)

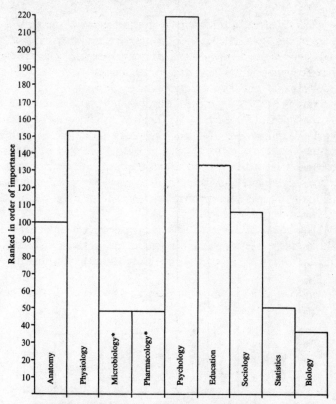

* Life sciences not ranked among the five most important subjects.
(Combinations of these subjects have been chosen by students as important)

can be seen between those subjects they rated as important in their own courses, and those they rated as important to the trained nurse. It should be noted that neither pharmacology nor microbiology was rated among the five most important subjects for the nurse tutor students, and yet both are considered important subjects for the trained nurse. The question to be addressed, therefore, is an important one. For since nurse tutors are responsible for the education of learners (the future trained nurses), who will provide tuition in these subjects for learners if they have not themselves been prepared to teach them during their own courses? This is clearly a matter of curricular and professional concern if those prepared specifically for

53

Figure 2.5: Nurse tutor students' choice of subjects in order of importance for the trained nurse (n = 324)

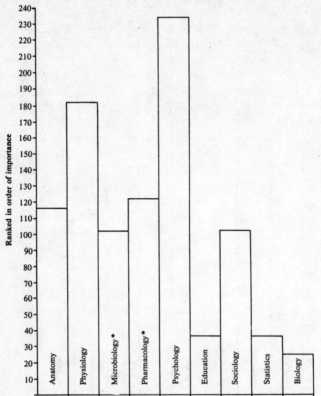

* (Combinations of these subjects have been chosen by the students, i.e. one respondent may have chosen more than one of these subjects as important.)

the purpose of teaching learners consider particular subjects of low priority in their own courses and yet rate the same subjects as important for the trained nurse. Moreover, the ranking of psychology as the most important subject for both groups (nurse tutor students and trained nurses) must be viewed with concern. There is now substantial evidence to suggest that the behavioural sciences are important to all nurses (Crow, 1976; Clarke, 1981; Wattley and Müller, 1983). However, it may be argued that the study of educational psychology on nurse tutor courses provides a limited, specialised background and does not prepare the nurse tutor students for the responsibility of teaching psychology after qualifying (Sheehan, 1981).

A perennial problem in nursing education is the acknowledged mixed ability of learners and the need for the development of appropriate strategies by tutors which will cater for the diverse needs of learners. It is important that appropriate teaching methods be used in order to present difficult concepts in as many different ways as possible to ensure learners' understanding and later ability to use the knowledge gained from their studies. Of the students surveyed in the sample, 80.9% were on one-year 'methods only' courses, and for them the development of varieties of teaching method is especially emphasised during their preparation. Respondents were accordingly asked to state the importance they attached to four types of teaching method in relation to (a) theory, and (b) practice, when teaching learners with varying levels of educational backgrounds. The results are presented in Table 2.2.

Table 2.2: Nurse tutor students' indication of the uses of specified teaching methods[a] in the teaching of theory and practice of nursing in relation to the life sciences ($n = 324$)

Teaching methods identified[a]	Group A ($n = 262$)		Group B ($n = 34$)		Group C ($n = 28$)	
	n	%	n	%	n	%
Group discussion						
Practice	206	78.6	27	79.4	20	71.4
Theory	204	77.9	20	58.8	23	82.1
Questioning techniques						
Theory	197	75.2	25	73.5	21	75.0
Practice	155	59.2	21	61.8	19	67.9
Simulations to encourage activity learning						
Practice	189	72.1	29	85.3	—	—
Theory	151	57.7	21	61.8	—	—
Project assignment						
Practice	185	70.6	26	76.5	19	67.9
Theory	152	58.0	15	44.1	13	46.4

[a] Chosen because they represent methods that demand an adequate knowledge base if the student is to use them effectively.

The results represent a combination of responses, as one respondent may have chosen any combination of the methods. Table 2.2 is important in terms of its implications for this study, since a concern with the practical application of theory is central to nursing education at all levels.

These methods demand an adequate knowledge base, and it is important for nurse tutors to possess that base and to be confident

about their ability to draw upon it. The use of these techniques
without a real understanding of the accompanying knowledge base
could constitute a real problem and, perhaps, one more source of
anxiety.

Anxiety in nurse tutor students

When all these factors are taken together, they represent a
formidable catalogue of problem areas and challenges for teachers
of nurses. The importance of anxiety and its effects on the individual
have been extensively reported in the literature. Much of this has
been concerned with patients' well-being (Hayward, 1975; Wilson-
Barnett, 1978; Boore, 1978). Learners' anxieties in relation to their
training have been reported by Birch (1979) and Parkes (1980). One
of the reasons for anxiety in learners found by Birch was the
discrepancy between what is taught in the school of nursing and the
reality of ward practice. This discrepancy is also evident in learners'
written examination answers and what they actually do when faced
with the reality of ward practice (Bendall, 1976). On the other hand,
Parkes's study reported clinical experiences on surgical wards as
being more stressful for learners than those on medical wards. She
notes the demands made upon technical skills and specific
knowledge which learners are required to demonstrate in the
performance of technical care.

Both learner anxiety and the demonstrable gap between theory
and practice have important implications for the education of nurse
tutors. At the same time, very little thought appears to have been
given to the anxieties which the teachers themselves might
experience. In the GNC survey (1975), it was found that all grades
of nurse teacher considered the conflict between education and
service as the most unsatisfactory aspect of their work as teachers.
In practice, this conflict is often translated into the broader issue of
theory and practice in which the possession or lack of knowledge
could be a crucial factor for the nurse teacher (Akinsanya, 1984).
In Table 2.2, respondents favoured the benefits of various teaching
methods in relation to practice, though the value of improving the
quality of theoretical learning and understanding also received
considerable emphasis.

Nevertheless, a question central to the present study remains, i.e.
the extent to which epistemiological problems affect those who are
being prepared to teach nursing. The life sciences provide a

Table 2.3: Nurse tutor students who felt concerned 'often' or 'always' about teaching the life sciences for the reasons shown (n = 324)

Possible causes of anxiety in nurse tutor students[a]	Group A (n = 262)		Group B (n = 34)		Group C (n = 28)	
	n	%	n	%	n	%
Lack of adequate knowledge of the subject myself	222	84.7	31	91.2	26	92.9
Attempting to simplify biological facts to learners	217	82.8	29	85.3	26	92.9
Having to rely on the medical model to explain biological aspects of nursing care	195	74.4	29	85.3	18	64.3
A shortage of books and teaching materials prepared by specialist nurses	180	68.7	27	79.4	26	92.9
Lack of access to patients while on teaching practice	155	59.2	25	73.5	8	28.6

[a]Combinations of these responses were stated by respondents.

knowledge base to which nurses can go directly for a relevant underpinning of much of their professional practice. Yet their reliance on such a knowledge presupposes the ability of those who teach nursing to understand this knowledge base in such a way that they are clear about its application in practice, and can transmit this to learners. The evidence reviewed in the literature survey suggests that at least five areas represent possible sources of anxiety for nurse tutor students. Respondents were asked how often they felt concerned in relation to each of the five areas. The results are shown in Table 2.3.

In the light of the evidence presented here, the following conclusions may be drawn.

(1) Nurse tutor students are, in general, well qualified educationally and professionally on entry to their courses. The possession of the Diploma in Nursing appears to be helpful in relation to an understanding of the role of the life sciences in their preparation. However, the exclusion of these subjects from one-year courses may be an undesirable condition and needs to be reviewed.

(2) The differences between the three types of course are matters of general rather than specific issues. The Group A course, by its nature of concentrated one-academic-year commitment, appears to be favoured by respondents. However, it should be

noted that part-time two-year courses are not only more effective in terms of the theory–practice link desired by the profession, but they are also more cost-effective and helpful to students. As noted earlier, the Briggs Report (1972) favoured this approach (Bosanquet and Clifton, 1973), and respondents on these courses have apparently found the arrangement satisfactory from the point of view of their domestic commitments.

(3) The overwhelming evidence suggests that the life sciences are not only important to the professional development of students, but are also seen to be so. For, irrespective of the type of course being attended, respondents were emphatic on the important role that a knowledge and an understanding of these sciences play in the performance of nursing functions. The views of nurse tutor students reflect a general professional approach which regards the possession of knowledge as important provided it is applied to practice. The life sciences emerge from this survey with a clear recognition of their usefulness and importance to the needs of learners and their future teachers. It is clear that institutional policies affect the way the students viewed the role of the subjects in their preparation. With the demise in 1982 of the Sister-Tutor Diploma of the University of London (STD) course, the issues raised by the formal exclusion of the life sciences from existing courses needs to be examined. The views of course directors will therefore be considered.

THE PREPARATION OF NURSE TUTORS: COURSE DIRECTORS' VIEWS

At the time of this study, 12 institutions offered courses for the preparation of teachers of nurses in England and Wales. These courses were approved by the GNC and validated either by universities or by the Council for National Academic Awards (CNAA). The courses for the preparation of teachers of nurses are of two kinds:

(1) Those preparing clinical teachers in either six months full time or one year part time. In the former case, the certificate is awarded by the RCN and it entitles the successful student to register with the GNC as a clinical nurse teacher (RCNT). The latter course is the City and Guilds Further Education Teachers'

Certificate (No. 730) or FETC. In this case, a successful candidate is registered as RCNT by the GNC if successful in Part A of the Diploma in Nursing of the University of London.

(2) Those preparing nurse tutors in two years full time for the STD — discontinued in 1982 — or the Diploma in Nursing Education (DipNEd) after a one-year full-time course or two years part time as described above.

Two main questions were addressed in the course directors' study.

(1) What are the general and specific (i.e. life-science-related) factors that determine the nature and purpose of nurse tutor preparation?

(2) What are the views of course directors on the contribution of the biological/life sciences to the preparation of nurse tutors?

Quantitative data obtained from the interview schedule covered:

(a) entrance requirements for the course, both educational and professional;

(b) formal teaching of the life sciences on the course and, if so, by whom;

(c) the importance of the life (biological) sciences in nurse tutor preparation to the teaching of the life sciences in their own courses;

(d) the effectiveness of the approach to the teaching of the biological sciences in the programme;

(e) whether or not the effectiveness is evaluated;

(f) teaching methods in use in their own courses;

(g) supervision of teaching practice and particularly of the biological content of lessons;

(h) liaison with schools of nursing, and schools' role in teaching practice both generally and in relation to the life sciences;

(i) library and other facilities.

Results of pre-coded responses by course directors in England and Wales are presented in Table 2.4. The findings may be summarised as follows:

(1) Eight of the twelve course directors qualified as nurse tutors through the Sister-Tutor Diploma of the University of London.

(2) Two course directors were non-nurses. Four courses were

Table 2.4: Pre-coded responses of course directors to questions on interview schedule (n = 12)

Item on interview schedule	Response of course directors	n
General course requirement	Professional experience as stipulated by GNC	10
	Passes in 2 GCE O levels	3
	Passes in 5 GCE O levels	7
	GCE A level desirable	1
Specific course requirement required	Passes in science subjects at O level	4
Other qualifications	DipN Part A required	8
	DipN Parts A and B required	8
	RCNT and JBCNS certificates	10
Minimum professional qualification required	SRN and RMN (separately)	9
	Dual (SRN/RMN/RSCN/RNMS)	1
Assumed knowledge of the biological sciences	Sufficient if passed Part A only	8
	Sufficient if passed DipN Parts A and B	2
Conduct of entrance test for teaching	To test general knowledge and aptitude	4
Biological sciences, nature of inclusion	Included in the course	2
	Excluded	8
	Through specialist lecturers	2
Participation of medical staff	Medical staff excluded	9
	Medical staff included	1
Teaching biological aspects	By non-specialist staff	5
	Taught by specialist staff	2
	Taught by nurse tutors	3
Teaching methods in use	Lecture	10
	Seminar	10
	Clinical involvement	2
	Group discussion	10
	Project assignments	8
	Tutorials	10
	Video recording and closed-circuit TV	10
Views on the importance of biological sciences in nurse tutor preparation	Very important	8
	Important	2
Effectiveness of the approach to the teaching of the biological sciences in the programme	Approach is effective	7
	Biological sciences not taught	3
Methods used in the evaluation of the use of the biological sciences in nurse tutor preparation	Effectiveness not evaluated	7
	Methods in use are effective	3
Involvement of students in ward-based teaching	Encouraged but not enforced	10

Table 2.4 *contd*

Supervision of students' teaching practice	By college and hospital staff	10
Supervision of biological contents of lessons	Difficult for non-nurse supervisors	10
Supervision of lessons	Before it is given by the student	8
Form of lesson supervision	Discussion of contents and offer of detailed comments	5
	Detailed written comments while lesson is being prepared	5
Average number of visits to students when on teaching practice	3 visits per term	3
	4 or more visits per term	7
Liaison with schools of nursing	Regularly — at least monthly	10
Is a formal report given by the school on each student at the end of teaching practice?	Yes — formal reports are given	10
Are specific references made to the teaching of biological sciences in such reports?	Yes — references are made to the students' teaching related to the biological sciences	5
	Normally a general report is issued	5
Library facilities for biological/medical and nursing subjects	Adequate and satisfactory	10
Provision of a separate library facility for the use of nurse tutor students in the departments	General library facilities are available and meet the needs of all students	10
Nursing journals regularly taken by the institution's libraries	*Nursing Times*	10
	Nursing Mirror	6
	Nursing Research	10
	Journal of Advanced Nursing	7
	International Journal of Nursing Studies	5
	Nursing Outlook	6

based in polytechnics, two in universities, two in teacher training colleges, two in technical colleges, one in a further education college, and one at the RCN.

(3) Three course directors would accept a minimum of two O levels provided professional qualifications and references were satisfactory. Nine required five O level passes.

(4) Eight institutions did not stipulate passes in science subjects, and four insisted on a science subject and England language.

(5) Nine courses would admit applicants with RMN or RNMS (Registered Mental Nurse and Registered Nurse for Mental Subnormality); three would do so with considerable reservation.

(6) Ten course directors would accept Part A of the Diploma in Nursing, but two insisted on both Parts A and B.

(7) Nine of the course directors accepted that the Diploma in Nursing provided adequate background knowledge of the life sciences for intending nurse tutors. Three considered the knowledge inadequate.

(8) Entrance tests were conducted in four institutions mainly for aptitude, literacy and numeracy. Eight course directors were not convinced of the usefulness of such tests.

(9) Two courses had a specific life science module, and ten completely excluded such specific input from their courses.

(10) Three of the course directors favoured the use of qualified nurse tutors with responsibility for linking the life sciences to nursing on their courses.

(11) Eleven course directors excluded medical participation in the preparation of nurse tutors, but medical participation was still central in the only course for the STD at the time of the survey.

(12) Three institutions specifically evaluated the use of the life sciences by students during the course, and five institutions specifically supervised lesson preparation in the life sciences. In general, all course directors used designated tutors in schools of nursing for regular but unobtrusive supervision of students when in the school of nursing.

(13) On average, six supervised visits were paid to each student by college staff during the academic session.

(14) All courses provided schools of nursing with standardised forms for the evaluation of student tutor teaching sessions. Seven course directors welcomed and encouraged comments from schools of nursing on the student tutors' use of the life sciences, and five were not particularly concerned about subject matter at all.

(15) Library facilities were viewed as adequate in all the established institutions, but one newly introduced course was dependent on a school of nursing for this. All institutions reported subscriptions to major nursing journals published in the United Kingdom.

The evidence indicates that all courses reflect the former GNC's stipulated entry requirement in terms of professional experience prior to undertaking the preparation as a nurse tutor. There are variations, however, in relation to the educational qualifications, with three institutions accepting 2 GCE O level passes. Although nine of the courses would accept a single registrable qualification, e.g. RMN, it was clear from the interviews that an applicant with such a qualification would be advised to consider future career development particularly as dual qualification could well be essential for career prospects.

On the whole, medical lectures are discouraged, with only one course retaining the medical contribution. As this was a two-year full-time course, the medical participation is a requirement of the syllabus in order to cover pathophysiology. The teaching of the life sciences thus becomes an important issue, and only in three courses are these taught by nurse tutors themselves. This has implications for the teaching practice supervision and particularly that of the biological contents or lessons. Because the teaching of the biological sciences is formally excluded from the majority of the courses, however, the need for such supervision and the evaluation of the effectiveness of the biological sciences approach to students' teaching was apparently being disregarded. It is interesting to note, however, that all course directors were vehement in their views that the development of a knowledge base in the life sciences is crucial to the development of nursing education.

Although these coded responses from the interview schedule represent quantifiable data from which inferences may be drawn, they are treated in this study as pointers to the underlying views of course directors, with all the elements of subjectivity implied in recorded interviews. There is nevertheless a strong suggestion in the data that the life sciences occupy what may be termed the 'hidden' aspect of the curriculum for the preparation of nurse tutors. Clearly, the use of the sciences is implicit in the coded responses whether or not formal exclusion of the subjects is an institutional policy. It is evident that course requirements vary between institutions, and the Diploma in Nursing (either Part A or Parts A and B) represents a major admission requirement to the nurse tutor course. It would also appear that the RCNT qualification and the JBCNS certificates are considered to be important background preparation for entry to nurse tutor courses.

A number of central issues were identified through content analysis and categorisation of themes using independent coders for the course directors' interviews. These were related to admission policy, educational backgrounds of applicants and professional issues such as the increasing admission of registered clinical teachers. Results from these qualitative analyses indicate that, for all the categorised themes, course directors were less influenced in their admission policies than would be expected from official views. This is a surprising finding, particularly because both the Diploma in Nursing and RCNT qualifications were repeatedly mentioned as essential admission requirements by course directors. As reported above, a large proportion of students surveyed possessed these two qualifications on admission. In effect, university/college requirements appear to be the most important influence on admission procedure followed by the possession of the Diploma in Nursing. The influence of other factors such as post-registration experience and the qualification as RCNT do not appear to be heavily weighted in admission procedures. Certainly, approval of post-registration experiences of applicants by the GNC (ENB) is compulsory, and that decision lies outside the control of course centres.

It may be inferred from this evidence that course directors are influenced by a number of factors of which college admission policy is the most influential. Nevertheless, there are other factors that are taken into consideration in the preparation of nurse tutors. Because of the overwhelming number of one-year full-time courses compared with the two-year full-time and two-year part-time courses (and the small number of course directors involved), a comparison could not be made between these courses. However, analysis of the transcribed materials suggests that five factors are important in nurse tutor preparation as viewed by the present study. These are:

(a) previous general education;
(b) general and specific professional qualifications;
(c) theory and application of the life sciences to nursing;
(d) knowledge base in life and behavioural sciences for nursing practice;
(e) application for nursing research.

The survey of course directors provided an opportunity to examine some of the issues that determine the nature and purpose of nurse tutor preparation. On a number of these issues, it was clear from the interviews that a trend towards the development of a nursing knowledge base in the life sciences seems to be emerging from these courses.

PERCEPTIONS AT THREE LEVELS

The summary of the empirical work presented in this chapter suggests that, at all three levels (learners, nurse tutor students and course directors), there are certain perceptions held in common.

(1) There is considerable agreement in the literature reviewed on the importance of the life sciences to the practising nurse demonstrating professional competence and delivering high-quality care — whatever the yardstick used to measure 'quality'. The role of the life sciences in professional development is, however, less clear, though there appears to be general agreement that a life sciences knowledge provides some of the reasons for actions in the performance of nursing tasks. This is, however, a very general statement whose implications (though acknowledged within the profession) do not seem to have informed course provision except in the most general way. The theory/practice link emerged from this study as being ill-defined and largely implicit in all areas of training. Thus it may be argued that the knowledge input remains theoretical, sterile and difficult, 'out there' rather than the *raison d'être* for nursing care. The majority of presently available textbooks in the life sciences reinforce this problem (Akinsanya, 1984).

(2) There is evidence of an emerging consensus about the desirability of a nursing model for nurse education, centred upon the concept of 'care', which might comprise:
(a) routine tasks involving skills and techniques rooted in the life sciences of anatomy, physiology, pharmacology and microbiology;
(b) decision-making within the limits of professional responsibility, which is crucially dependent upon a full understanding of the reason for every action, or non-action. These, in turn, are also essentially rooted in the life sciences of anatomy, physiology, pharmacology and microbiology;
(c) interpersonal relations, which depend upon an understanding of the reasons for action, which lie mainly in the social/behavioural sciences.

There is also some evidence of anxiety about the life sciences in both learners and nurse tutor students. Learners' anxiety appears to centre upon what they see as the ineffectiveness of the teaching of the life sciences in their training; and on the 'difficulty' of what they have to learn (partly because of the fact that largely experimental subjects are taught theoretically, partly because they have difficulty in seeing the relevance of the theoretical knowledge transmitted in lectures for the tasks they are being trained to perform in the wards, and partly because they are themselves ill-prepared to meet the educational challenges of these subjects in nurse education). It is particularly important to note that learners today are better educated and better able to cope with the theoretical aspects of their work and that they might also become frustrated by a stultifying exposure to lectures with little explicit relevance, taught by teachers with little demonstrable confidence in their ability to handle that relevance adequately because of their own perceived (and sometimes real) lack of understanding.

The difficulty perceived by learners at all stages of training in the study of the life sciences constitutes an important finding. The performance of a wide range of nursing procedures was perceived as dependent upon a knowledge of the life sciences, and, in particular, life-threatening situations for the patient were perceived as those in which a lack of knowledge of the appropriate life science in the nurse could be dangerous for the patient (e.g. care of the unconscious patient, and procedures which may involve invasion of the physical body space).

It is important to note, however, that an *understanding* of the reasons for nursing action, i.e. of the appropriate knowledge base, was perceived as being equally important, although learners' perceptions were perhaps coloured by their own immediate experiences on the wards. It would seem, however, that the relationships between the theoretical underpinning of nursing actions, and the realities of the practical application of this knowledge in clinical situations (in situations for which they will be individually responsible) remain an area of considerable uncertainty and a major source of learner anxiety.

Nurse tutor students also felt concerned about their own preparation in these sciences, especially in relation to their ability to teach them in learners (only 30 per cent of the respondents felt adequately prepared to teach them). This concern is likely to be exacerbated when confronting academically able learners with solid achievements in physics, chemistry and biology at A level.

Students on one-year courses expressed concern about their lack of access to patients on teaching practice, clearly an important means of linking theory with practice. Although course directors reported the use of a variety of techniques such as simulations in training nurse tutors, the effective use of these techniques is likely to be dependent upon the quality of the users' knowledge base. This applies both to nurse tutor training and to their use of these techniques in their own teaching as a supplement to, or a substitute for, teaching on the wards.

These are important findings with many implications for future research and for curriculum development. They offer some contrast, too, to course directors' perceptions. Although the latter perceive the life sciences as crucial in the preparation of nurse tutors, the reality of their official concern is the preparation of an adequate number of teachers for the needs of the profession, and one-year methods-only courses seem the obvious solution. As a result, they have to rely on an assumption that an appropriate level of knowledge and understanding is already available to nurse tutor students on entry to training, by virtue of their previous success in the Diploma in Nursing course.

Interestingly, course directors perceive a shift in the knowledge base of nursing from the life to the behavioural sciences. Yet there appears to be no desire to reverse such a shift in spite of the admitted consequences of inadequate tuition in the life sciences for learners. Indeed course directors were vehement about the important role of these subjects in nursing education, and saw the role of nurse tutors in their transmission as pivotal to safe practice. Yet ideal and reality appear poles apart, and institutional and professional demands are evidently met pragmatically. When the two conflict, compromise seems inevitable, with the result that the requirement of the nursing profession for tutors knowledgeable in the life sciences and able to transmit such knowledge in classroom and clinical areas, though recognised, appears to be subservient to institutional policy.

As we have seen, this situation is not helped by the fact that teaching practice supervision is often carried out by college staff without qualifications in the biological/life sciences who could clearly provide neither help with content in lesson preparation, nor an assessment of the accuracy of the lesson content, however competent to judge teaching ability they may be. It seems possible that more benefits would accrue from the closer involvement of schools of nursing in teaching practice. It is the specificity of the content of teaching that also calls into question the tendency to treat nurse tutor students as one among several professional groups within a methods-only course, a tendency that should be re-examined.

The study arose from the researcher's long-term observation that nursing, dependent as it has been on a largely medically orientated practice, has probably missed several opportunities to develop its own knowledge base, particularly in the life sciences. In the intervening two decades since this concern was first experienced, much has changed in nursing education. The approach in this study, which looked at the triangle of learners–tutors–course directors perspectives, exposed a number of problems with considerable curricula implications in relation to the learning, teaching and application of the life sciences in nursing education. (It is worth noting that the issues may be more acute for the life than for the behavioural sciences. The latter inform nurses about people and their behaviour under varying circumstances including stressful situations. It could be argued that the life sciences, on the other hand, mainly inform nursing practice in so far as they relate to the specific tasks involved in nursing care.)

A BIONURSING MODEL FOR TEACHING THE LIFE SCIENCES IN NURSE EDUCATION

Whatever conceptions qualified nurses may have of it, professional autonomy depends in part on what is taught, how it is learnt, the clarity of the learner's understanding and the judgements involved in its application in practice. All these issues can be examined by the use of the model, and at every stage of course planning in the life sciences it would seem that the model provides a means of delineating essential information for inclusion in the syllabus. Though as yet untested, it seems possible that the use of the model will also be helpful in ensuring transfer both vertically (as between simple and complex concepts) and laterally (in application in practice).

It would be hard, in the light of the evidence presented here, to dispute the views of learners and nurse tutor students that the teaching and learning of the life sciences currently present them with difficult educational problems. It would seem that course directors have an ambivalent attitude towards the inclusion of the life sciences in their courses. Indeed, although they vehemently assert their relevance and importance to the preparation of nurse tutors, they nevertheless push the responsibility for ensuring their appropriate input to pre-tutor courses. However, there are increasing grounds for questioning such an approach, not least of which is the evident anxiety of learners and nurse tutors whose professional practice depends, for the most part, on a sound grasp of knowledge derived from these sciences.

Certainly, the analytical problems are considerable, because the current nursing syllabus does not appear to encourage nurse educators to approach the teaching of the life sciences within a framework in which concepts and terms from these subjects are seen first and foremost as the legitimate vocabulary of nursing rather than as ideas borrowed from medicine. A *bionursing* link, because it may encourage the nurse to look directly at the roots rather than the branches of the life sciences and their application to nursing care, could lead to a better understanding of the reasons for their application, to greater professional competence and to enhanced patient care and welfare.

REFERENCES

Adams, W.E. and Taylor, D.W. (eds) (1974) *Gowland and Cairney's anatomy and physiology for nurses.* N.M. Peryer, Christchurch, New Zealand

Akinsanya, J.A. (1984) Development of a nursing knowledge base in the life sciences: problems and prospects. *International Journal of Nursing Studies, 21* (3), 221–7

Annett, J. (1971) *Task analysis.* HMSO, London (cited in L.B. Curzon (1980) *Teaching in further education: an outline of principles and practice,* 2nd edn, Cassell, London

Baldwin, S. (1983) Nursing models in special hospitals. *Journal of Advanced Nursing, 8* (6), 473–6

Bendall, E. (1976) Learning for reality. *Journal of Advanced Nursing, 1,* 3–9

Bendall, E. and Raybould, E. (1969) *History of the General Nursing Council for England and Wales, 1919–1969.* H.K. Lewis, London

Birch, J. (1979) The anxious learners. *Nursing Mirror, 148* (6), 17–22

Boore, J. (1978) *A prescription for recovery.* RCN, London

Bosanquet, N. and Clifton, R. (1973) Briggs: the context (3). Nursing work: some impressions. *Nursing Times, Occasional Papers, 69* (21) and *69* (22)

Briggs, A. (1972) *Report of the Committee on Nursing,* Cmnd 5115. HMSO, London

Chinn, P.L. (1983) Nursing theory development: where we have been and where we are going. In N.L. Chaska (ed.) *The nursing profession: a time to speak.* McGraw-Hill, London

Clarke, M. (1981) Two aspects of psychology and their applications to nursing. In J.P. Smith (ed.) *Nursing science in nursing practice.* Butterworth, London

Cox, C. (1982a) Frontiers of nursing in the 21st century: lessons from the past and present for future directions in nursing education. *International Journal of Nursing Studies, 19* (1), 1–9

Cox, C. (1982b) 'The seeds of time' — or the future of nurse education. *Nurse Education Today, 2* (6), 5–10

Crow, R.A. (1976) A fresh look at psychology in nursing. *Journal of Advanced Nursing, 1* (1), 51–62

Davis, B.D. (ed.) (1983a) *Research into nurse education.* Croom Helm, London

Davis, B.D. (1983b) A repertory grid study of formal and informal aspects of student nurse training. Unpublished PhD thesis, University of London

Demaree, R. (1961) Development of training equipment planning information (cited in K.U. Smith (1966) *Cybernetic principles of learning and education design,* Holt, Rinehart & Winston, New York

Edney, P. (1972) *A systems analysis of training.* Pitman, London

Faulkner, A. (1980) Communication and the nurse. *Nursing Times Occasional Papers, 76* (21), 93–5

Fitts, P. (1965) Factors in complex skill training, in R. Glaser (ed.) *Training research and education.* Wiley, New York

General Nursing Council for England and Wales (1975) *Educational survey.* General Nursing Council, London

General Nursing Council for England and Wales (1977) *Syllabus of subjects for examination for the Certificate of General Nursing,* General Nursing Council, London

Greaves, F. (1979) Teaching nurses in clinical settings. *Nursing Mirror* (Supplement), *148* (8), i–viii

Hainsworth, M. (1936) *Modern professional nursing.* Caxton, London

Hayward, J.C. (1975) *Information — a prescription against pain. The study of nursing care,* Series 2, No. 5. RCN, London

Hayward, J.C. and Lelean, S.R. (1982) Nursing research, in P. Allan and M. Jolley (eds) *Nursing, midwifery and health visiting since 1900.* Faber & Faber, London, pp. 196–214

Holford, H.K. (1981) Requirements for nursing. *Nursing Times, 77* (3), 113

Holmes, B. (1972) Nursing as a profession: a comparative approach. *Nursing Times, 68* (21), 655–6

Inman, U. (1975) *Towards a theory of nursing care,* Studies of Nursing Care, Series No. 2. RCN, London

Macleod Clark, J. and Hockey, L. (1979) *Research for nursing. A guide for the enquiring nurse.* HM & M Publishers, London

McCarthy, W.H. (1972) Egoistical specialists and nursing students. *Nursing Times, 68* (3), 41–4

McFarlane, J. (1977) Developing a theory of nursing: the relation of theory to practice, education and research. *Journal of Advanced Nursing, 2,* 261–70

Nolan, R.J. (1973) The development of teaching methods in human biology within nurse training schools, unpublished MEd thesis, University of Manchester

Parkes, K.R. (1980) Occupational stress among student nurses — 1. A comparison of medical and surgical wards. *Nursing Times Occasional Papers, 76* (25), 113–16

Peterson, C.J.W. (1983) Overview of issues in nursing education, in N.L. Chaska (ed.), *The nursing profession: a time to speak.* McGraw-Hill, New York and London

Phillipson, P.A.J. (1982) Letter to the Editor, *Nursing Mirror, 155* (4), 36

Roper, N., Logan, W.W. and Tierney, A.J. (1981) *Learning to use the process of nursing.* Churchill Livingstone, Edinburgh

Sheahan, J. (1981) Developing teaching skills. *Nursing Focus, 3* (3), 543–7

Starck, P. (1984) Realism in nursing curricula. *Nursing Outlook, 32* (4)

Wattley, L. and Muller, D.J. (1983) Psychology and nursing: the case for an empirical approach. *Journal of Advanced Nursing, 8* (2), 107–10

Wilson-Barnett, J. (1978) Factors influencing patients' emotional reactions to hospitalization. *Journal of Advanced Nursing, 3,* 221–9

Wilson, K.J.W. (1975) *A study of biological sciences in relation to nursing.* Churchill Livingstone, Edinburgh

3

Mathematics for Nursing

S.E.B. Pirie

INTRODUCTION

The traditional role of the nurse has undergone dramatic changes over the last couple of decades. The image of 'a girl with a vocation to tend the sick' is no longer adequate to describe the nurse who must now work with rapidly advancing technology, scientific knowledge of increasing complexity, and an ever-changing range of powerful drugs. Listening to patients, understanding their problems and counselling them as well as ministering to their physical needs are of course still all vital parts of nursing, but so too is an ability to calculate and communicate mathematical and scientific information with accuracy. Unfortunately we cannot assume that this latter ability is automatically present in today's nurses. In fact anecdotes, reports and research results would indicate otherwise.

What little reported detail there is of nursing errors is largely confined to drug administration. Events such as the death of a child from an overdose of digoxin may be widely reported, but what evidence is there of less dramatic nursing errors? It is hard to assess the size of the problem at a non-fatal level, but a study in 1979, by G.C. Brown in Michigan, produced the following breakdown of errors in drug administration: wrong dose 20%; wrong drug 17%; omission 15%; wrong rate of infusion 13%; wrong route 11%; wrong time 11%; other errors (wrong patient, duplication of dose, etc.) 13%. Of these errors, wrong dose and wrong rate of infusion, together giving 33% of the total, are likely to be mathematical errors. The number of drug dosage errors varies from one research project to another (Barker and McConnell, 1962; Apple, 1976) but this is natural when it is remembered that only reported errors can be evaluated. In a special observational study Barker and McConnell

(1962) recorded that of over 51 000 medication errors observed, only 56 were detected by the nurse and of those only 36 were reported!

An alternative method of error assessment is via simulational testing. Williamson and White (1974) reported that 1 in 24 practising nurses failed to reach an acceptable minimum level of ability in drug administration due 'to a lack of competence in dosage calculation'. In 1979 Perlstein *et al.* reported on their work with paediatric staff in an intensive care unit. They found a mean error rate of 24% and '56% of the errors tabulated would have resulted in administered doses ten times greater or ten times less than the ordered dose'. This horrific tale was borne out by the second phase of a study into the deficiencies in basic mathematical skills among nurses (Pirie, 1983a), to be described in greater detail later in this chapter.

Although possibly the most obvious, drug dosage is by no means the only area in which mathematical skills are involved. Mathematical errors have been reported in such widely differing tasks as infant feeding and graphical recording. Wilkinson *et al.* (1973) reported on an experiment to discover how accurately dried milk powder was measured out for infant feeds and showed 100% variation in one case and consistent over-concentration of powder in all cases. One of the prime purposes of graphical recording is to present, at a glance, a visual picture of the information gathered. Pirie (1983b) discusses one incident, among many, in which the scales on a printed diabetic chart had been altered by a nurse in such a way as to totally distort the impression of dramatic change in urine-sugar levels. The research reported above indicates some of the areas in which errors have been recorded. To investigate the situation more deeply it is necessary first to try to answer the question: what mathematics is it that a nurse should know?

TAXONOMY OF NURSING MATHEMATICS

In 1981 a study was undertaken to compile a comprehensive list of nursing mathematics. In order to ensure that all the possible areas of mathematics used in nursing were included in this list, the study was based on three job-analysis projects (Scottish Home and Health Department, 1967; Williams, 1977; Moores and Moult, 1979). An observation schedule of tasks was built up and these tasks were categorised as 'unlikely', 'possible' and 'definite' sources of

Figure 3.1: Taxonomy of nursing mathematics

Topic	Upper Bound (U) and Mastery Level (M)	Uses (common examples)	Behavioural Objectives To be able to —
A Addition of whole numbers	1204 + 359 (U,M)	Fluid balance chart	add integers of up to 4 digits
B Subtraction of whole numbers	1320 − 575 (U,M)	Fluid balance chart	subtract integers of up to 4 digits
C Multiplication of whole numbers	125 × 4184 (U,M)	Convert calories to joules (1C = 4184 J) Weight related drugs, paediatric feeds, etc.	multiply integers of up to 4 digits
D Division with whole numbers	925 ÷ 125 (U,M)	Drug doses: 925 mg available as 125 mg/ml (From 25 mg/kg, weight = 37kg)	divide integers of up to 4 digits by integers 1–9 and multiples of 5
E Addition of fractions	$\frac{1}{2} + \frac{3}{8}$ (U,M)	Several injections of the same drug: Drug available as 1 mg in 5 ml. Mr X needs $\frac{2}{5}$ ml; Mr Y, $\frac{4}{5}$ ml; Mr Z, $\frac{3}{5}$ ml. Total $\frac{9}{5}$ ml = $1\frac{4}{5}$ ml => need 2×5 ml ampoules	add fractions with simple or common denominators, recognising equivalence
F Multiplication of fractions	$1\frac{1}{2} \times \frac{3}{5}$ (U,M)	$7\frac{1}{2}$ units of 40 strength insulin $= 7\frac{1}{2} \times \frac{1}{40} = \frac{5}{2} \times \frac{1}{40}$ ml	multiply mixed fractions with simple denominators, recognising equivalence
G Addition of decimals	10.26 + 3.055 (U,M)	Total energy in diet = 41.84J + 28.05 J. Paediatric feeds, expected weight gain, etc.	add decimals of up to 3 decimal places
H Subtraction of decimals	4.05 − 3.965 (U,M)	Weight gain of baby = 4.05 kg − 3.96 kg. Special diets	substract decimals of up to 3 decimal places
I Multiplication of decimals	0.725 × 1.32 (U)	Drug dose 0.75g, available 1g in 0.5 ml dose = 0.75 × 0.5 ml	multiply a decimal by an integer with up to 3 figures
	0.725 × 132 (M)	Drug doses normally available as × mg per y ml where y is an integer	

J Division of decimals	26.4 ÷ 75 (U,M)	Drug dose 62.5 mg, available 25 mg in 1 ml dose = $\frac{62.5}{25}$ ml	divide a decimal by the integers 1–9 and multiples of 5
K Division by decimals	0.45 ÷ 0.6 (U,M)	Drug dose 0.45 mg, available 0.6 mg in 1 ml dose = $\frac{0.45}{0.6}$ ml	divide a decimal by a single digit decimal
L Converting fractions to decimals	$\frac{5}{8}$ = (0.625) (U,M)	Particularly paediatric work. Injection dose = $\frac{2}{5}$ ml = 0.4 (Convert to use syringe)	understand that quantities commonly accepted as fractions still mean 'division' and are a simple case of D
M Converting decimals to fractions	1.25 = $(1\frac{1}{4})$ (U,M)	Drug dose = 1.25 = $1\frac{1}{4}$ tablets	convert '×.25', '×.5', '×.75' to fractions, where x is an integer
N Percentage	20% of 800 (U,M)	Solutions. 2 litres of 10% Dextrose contain $\frac{10}{100}$ × 2 l dextrose. Urine-sugar levels — percentages used as a label. Drug doses	calculate simple percentages
O Ratio problems	x mg required of a solution 1 to 5 or a solution 2 mg $\left[\begin{array}{c}\text{per}\\ \text{in}\end{array}\right]$ 3 ml (U,M)		calculate drug doses from a doctor's prescription
P Use of S.I. units	g mega (U) l kilo mol unit m milli J micro Pa g muga (M) l kilo unit m milli J micro	Convert 0.025 mg to micrograms All hospital measurements now in S.I. units, but Pascals and moles less frequently encountered than the others	work accurately with the S.I. units most frequently encountered

Figure 3.1 *contd*

Topic	Upper Bound (U) and Master Level (M)	Uses (Common Examples)	Behavioural Objectives To be able to—
Q Using formulae	Word formulae of form $A = \dfrac{B + C(D + E)}{F}$ (U) Word formulae of type $A \times \dfrac{C}{B}$ or $A \times B + C \times D$ (M) and selection of values from extra data	Expected weight = Birth weight + (Age in weeks − 2) in kg × normal weight gain in kg Drug doses, food requirements etc. The more complex formulae occur in specialist departments	calculate, using a formula expressed in words, infant feeds, fluid requirement, expected weight gains, drug doses, etc.
R Use of tables	S.I./Imperial (U,M) conversions Age/Normal weight gain	Most frequently used for communication with patients: 55.25 kg = 8 stone $9\frac{1}{2}$ lb Paediatric progress assessment	obtain information, convert S.I. ↔ imperial units from printed tables
S Meaning of Indices	Understand the (U) change between $a \times 10^y$ and $z \times 10^y$ and $z \times 10^p$ Meaning of $a \times 10^y$ (M)	Path. Lab. report 'Red cell count = 4.5×10^{12}' The nurse is usually the first person to see the path. lab. reports and therefore carries the responsibility of alerting the doctor if necessary	understand scientific reports on patients; information usually given in standard form
T Meaning of decimal place	$0.1 > 0.07$ (U,M)	Safety in estimation and accuracy in calculation Known adult dose 0.05 mg implies child's dose of 0.25 mg has been miscalculated	know the meaning of digits in various decimal places

U Making and filling in tables	Intensive care (U,M) ¼ hourly record	record information in an appropriate printed table
	See fluid balance chart	
V Plotting graphs	Multi-graph and (U,M) Diabetic graph	record information on a graph with scales already determined
	temp, blood-pressure, pulse, respiration, urine-sugar	
W Interpreting graphs	Paediatric I.C. (U,M) graph. Judge weight against a standard weight graph	read information off a graph and form judgements from these readings
	Alert doctor to significant change in temperature	
X Addition of negative numbers	1.2 + −0.3 (non-essential)	add +ve and −ve simple decimals
	Combining lens strengths in eye out-patients department (U)	

mathematical activity. The schedule was used in a wide variety of wards selected from three large hospitals to ensure that all the tasks were observed several times. Once confirmed, the 'unlikely' tasks, such as flower arranging, were deleted from the list. The remaining tasks were observed over a three-month period, and the 150 ward staff involved were invited to comment on any tasks which they felt were relevant. It must be emphasised at this point that the list was to contain the mathematics that a nurse needs on the job. For this reason statistics has not been included, although it is obviously a desirable area of understanding for those wishing to gain from their reading of reported research.

The mathematics required in each task was analysed and a detailed questionnaire was completed by 18 school of nursing tutors from two schools, with a view to establishing the upper bounds, or most difficult examples, of each skill which a nurse would be likely to meet.

The observation lists together with the questionnaires were used to compile a taxonomy of nursing mathematics with defined mastery levels and upper bounds for each topic. Figure 3.1 lists the topics (in column 1) with examples of the type of calculations involved (in column 2) and indications of areas of nursing where such topics occur (in column 3), and presents the behavioural objectives related to each topic which every practitioner needs to attain in order to nurse effectively and safely (in column 4). The examples given in the second column are at two levels. Those labelled U (upper bound) indicate a most difficult calculation within a particular topic which a nurse is likely to encounter. Those labelled M (mastery level) are typical of the level of mathematics which the nurse normally encounters and at which she should have mastery of the topic. The interesting feature of this list is that in the majority of areas the upper bounds and mastery levels are identical.

The value of this taxonomy is that it gives a comprehensive list of the mathematical topics in which any aspiring nurse should be competent, and can therefore be used as a basis for assessing relevant mathematical ability in nurses.

WHAT DO NURSES ALREADY KNOW?

In order to decide what should be taught to prospective nurses, it is necessary first to ascertain what they already know. Three factors which affect the mathematical abilities of those entering the profession must be borne in mind. First, the majority of entrants are still female and there is substantial research (Cockcroft Committee, 1982) demonstrating the fact that, for whatever reasons, girls are on the whole less good at mathematics than boys. Secondly, the problem of limited transfer is relevant (Ausubel, 1968; Gage and Berliner, 1979), Skills learned in one area, in this case 'school mathematics', are frequently not automatically applied in a different context such as drug calculation. Thirdly, students may be suffering from a considerable degree of forgetfulness since they may have ceased doing any mathematics two or, in the case of mature students, more years prior to starting their training. Their perception, therefore, of what they can do may be based on outdated memories.

With these considerations in mind, the compilation of the taxonomy was followed by the construction of a test to ascertain which of the mathematical topics were causing problems for nurses. The test was given to learners since it had already been shown that problems certainly existed among nurses, and the simplest place to do large-scale testing and to introduce remediation is during training. The intention was to use the test results to furnish answers to questions such as 'What mathematics can they not do?', and 'How extensive are the problems?' Prior to sitting the test, learners were asked to give certain biographical details and to assess their own abilities in the given topics. With this extra information it was hoped to discover factors that would allow the identification of those learners likely to have difficulties.

The objectives of the test were thus four-fold:

(1) to discover the number of learners having difficulty with some area of mathematics;
(2) to rate the difficulty for the learners of the topics;
(3) to determine whether certain biographical factors could be used to determine those learners 'at risk';
(4) to compare learners' own perceived difficulties with their actual performance.

Although the qualifying examinations for nurses are national, there exists considerable variation between schools of nursing in terms of entry requirements, social and geographical recruiting areas, and environments for clinical experience. Four schools were chosen to represent as far as possible a broad range of learners. Those taking part were:

(a) a small school requiring the minimum entry qualifications and recruiting mainly from the local area;

(b) a medium-sized school requiring more than minimum entry standard and recruiting approximately 60% of its learners locally;

(c) a large school requiring high entry standards and recruiting approximately 40% locally;

(d) a large, prestigious school, training for specialist paediatric nursing, stipulating mathematics O level at grade A, B or C among its high entry requirements, and recruiting internationally.

From these schools nearly 600 learners in 22 groups were asked to complete the test. The self-assessment section of the test presented the candidates with a topic list together with examples of the relevant calculations, and required them to rate their expected performance from 1 to 4 using the following criteria:

1: Easy means: could do it in my head
might need a scrap of paper
sure of how to do it
confident the answer will be right

2: Fairly easy means: could probably do it given time
would definitely need paper or tables
reasonably sure I know how to do it
fairly confident the answer would be right

3: Difficult means: would need some help
would need a calculator
not quite sure how to do it
would need to check with someone

4: Impossible means: could not do it
would get someone to do it for me

The questions in the mathematics test were constructed in such a way that their solutions could also be marked from 1 to 4 on the same criteria. Most questions consisted of two parts and were scored along the lines of the scheme outlined below. The comments given in brackets are those on which the learners based their self-assessment of ability.

Score 1 if:
whole question correct ('sure of how to do it')
> with no written working ('do it in my head')
> with trivial written working ('might need a scrap of paper')

Score 2 if:
whole question correct, but
> with heavy working ('definitely need paper')
> with erroneous attempts ('probably do it given time')
> or there is a slip in one part ('fairly confident')

Score 3 if:
> one part fundamentally wrong ('not quite sure how to do it')
> one part omitted ('need some help/calculator')
> or there is a slip in both parts ('need someone to check it')

Score 4 if:
whole question wrong ('could not do it')
> or omitted ('get someone else to do it'/'don't know how to
> begin')

What is the significance of a 2-, 3- or 4-score in nursing terms? It is clearly impossible to quantify the danger inherent in a mathematical error without precise knowledge of the context in which it occurs. In general terms, however, a 2-score indicates that under pressure a usually accurate nurse might make a mistake. The real problem with 3- and 4-scores occurs if there is a mismatch between actual and perceived ability. If the nurse *knows* she does not know how to perform a calculation, then she will seek help. If, on the other hand, she is not aware of her failings or has unfounded confidence in her mathematical skills, then in certain circumstances there could be serious consquences for her patients.

The results of the mathematical test are given in Figure 3.2 in terms of rounded percentages of learners achieving each score for each topic, and indicate clearly the proportions of learners with difficulties. Unfortunately question V, on graph plotting, threw up some unexpected errors and these created problems with allocation of the 1- to 4-scores. Question W, on interpretation, was affected by these errors and so these two topics were not considered in any of the subsequent analyses.

As can be seen, topics such as A, B, C, D, G, I, R and U were causing few learners to fail, although only 19% of the learners actually achieved a mastery score in I, decimal multiplication. Mastery scores in other topics such as ratio, SI units and decimal division were also very low.

Figure 3.2: Achievement score distribution

Topic	Percentages of scores						
	1	2	3	4			
A	71	25	4	0	+		
B	45	41	13	1	−	} Integers	
C	42	45	12	1	×		
D	48	15	35	2	÷		
E	47	19	20	14	+	} Fractions	
F	22	23	11	44	×		
G	67	25	8	1	+		
H	22	33	28	17	−		
I	19	46	29	6	×	} Decimals	
J	20	12	47	21	÷		
K	23	18	8	51	÷		
L	25	10	30	35	} Decimals ⟷ fractions		
M	55	5	11	29			
N	53	14	2	31	Percentage		
O	12	3	44	41	Ratio		
P	5	22	37	36	SI units		
Q	43	6	16	35	Formulae		
R	58	30	4	7	Printed tables		
S	35	3	11	51	Indices		
T	30	2	8	10	Place value		
U	91	2	1	6	Tabular recording		
V	34	18	19	29	Plot	} graphs	
W	18	4	13	65	Interpret		
X	25	11	22	42	Negative numbers		

Three different methods were used to rate the topics in order of difficulty. Only a score of 1 indicated that the learner had mastery at the required level in that topic, and so the topics were first ordered by the total number failing to achieve a 1-score. Secondly, the topics were ranked according to the number of learners getting a 4-score, and finally, since a score of 3 was also a cause for alarm, the topics were ranked by those achieving a 3- or 4-score. Table 3.1 gives the 'top ten' by each ranking method.

Seven topics (SI units, ratio, decimal division, decimal/fraction conversion, indices, fractional multiplication and negative numbers) can be seen to be ranked among the top ten by all three methods. In addition, nearly a third of the sample completely failed the percentage questions, and over one-half had problems with substitution into word formulae.

Table 3.1: Topics ranked for difficulty

Rank	Lack of mastery (%)		Complete failure (%)		Experiencing difficulty (%)	
1	P	95	K,S	51	O	85
2	O	88	—		P	73
3	I	81	F	44	J	68
4	J	80	X	42	L	65
5	F,H	78	O	41	X	64
6	—		P	36	S	62
7	K	77	L,Q	35	K	59
8	L,X	75	—		F	55
9	—		N	31	Q	51
10	S	65	M	29	H	45

WHO NEEDS HELP?

Reference to Figure 3.1 reveals that these topics occur in such everyday tasks as calculating drug doses, reading laboratory results and dealing with solutions. Word formulae occur particularly in paediatric and neonatal work, and in this area even small errors can be dangerous. SI units, of course, affect almost everything the nurse does.

It is evident from these results that large numbers of learners have problems with some areas of mathematics. Can these learners be easily identified? One possible focus for consideration is public examination qualifications. Alternatively, stage of training or status as pupil or student may be relevant. Simplest of all, do those with problems know their weaknesses? Details from the biographical survey were analysed against test results to investigate whether there was any correlation between test performance and pre-entry qualifications, year of training, status or self-assessment score.

As might be expected, there was a connection between A level, O level, CSE, no mathematical qualification and the respective test scores. This is illustrated in Figure 3.3. As can be seen, the higher the external qualification, whether in mathematics or in a related subject such as physics, the larger the proportion of candidates achieving a 1-score. What is also evident from Figure 3.4, however, is that even A-level mathematics does not guarantee mastery in all the necessary mathematics for nursing. Two factors must also be

Figure 3.3: Test grades related to GCE and CSE qualifications

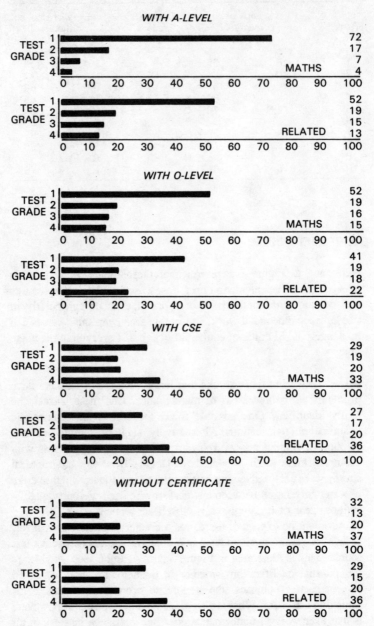

Figure 3.4: Test grades related to status: student or pupil

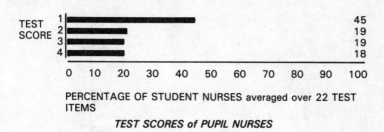

TEST SCORES of STUDENT NURSES

PERCENTAGE OF STUDENT NURSES averaged over 22 TEST ITEMS

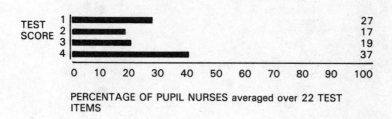

TEST SCORES of PUPIL NURSES

PERCENTAGE OF PUPIL NURSES averaged over 22 TEST ITEMS

borne in mind: the mathematics required is only a small subset of the O-level syllabus, and mathematical ability is only one of a number of qualities required of a prospective nurse. To require A-level mathematics for entry to training would be totally inappropriate.

Consideration of the test scores in relation to year of training showed that there was no significant correlation, and so it cannot be assumed that the learners will just 'pick up' the skills they need as they go through their training. There was a correlation between status and test score, with the students as a group being rated better at nursing mathematics than the pupils. Figure 3.4, however, illustrates the fact that less than half the students were achieving the necessary mastery levels.

The easiest way of helping learners with their problems would be to recommend suitable texts or tutorial time to those who ask for them. This is only an effective way of dealing with the situation if learners are themselves aware of their problems. Figure 3.5 demonstrates very clearly that this is not the case. The white

85

Figure 3.5: Self-assessed and actual fail scores on 22 topics

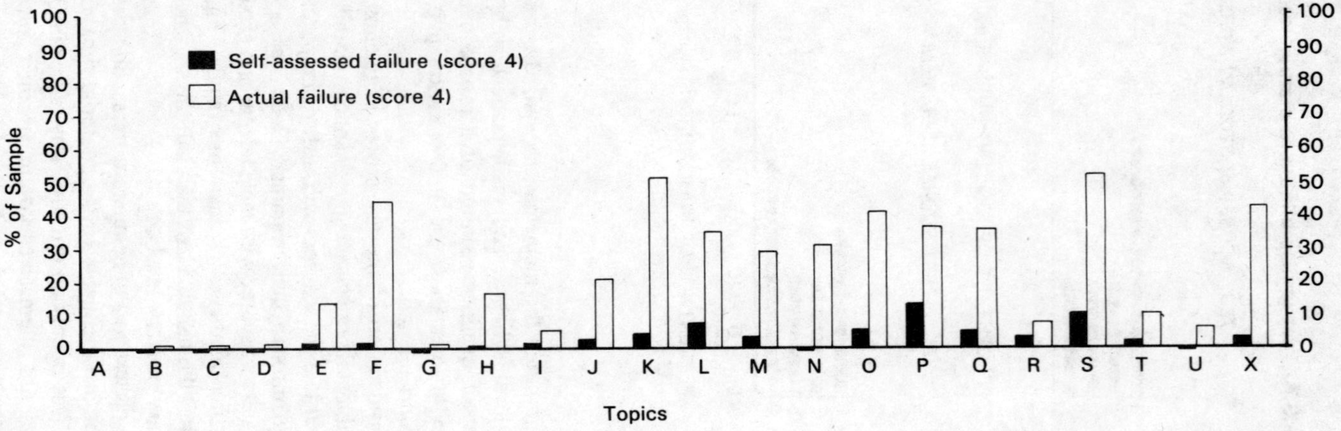

Self-assessed failure (score 4)

Actual failure (score 4)

% of Sample

Topics

Figure 3.6: Comparison of achieved and assessed scores

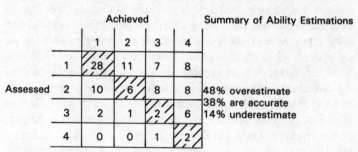

Assessed	Achieved 1	2	3	4	Summary of Ability Estimations
1	28	11	7	8	
2	10	6	8	8	48% overestimate
3	2	1	2	6	38% are accurate
4	0	0	1	2	14% underestimate

columns indicate the number of learners who failed in each topic, and the black columns indicate those who predicted failure. In every topic except A, B and C, learners were overestimating their abilities and would therefore be unlikely to seek the help they needed. In fact the learners were not even consistent in their self-assessment. Figure 3.6 shows the comparison between achieved and assessed scores and reveals that only 38% of the responses of the self-assessment task were accurate. A scrutiny of individuals' self-assessed scores revealed that the great majority of the learners did not even consistently over- or underestimate their ability. As much research has shown (for example, Cowan, 1975; Morton and Macbeth, 1977; Daines, 1978), this is not a phenomenon peculiar to nurses, and heed must be paid to Huckabay's injunction (1981) that teachers should 'rely more on objective tests to measure the entering behaviour of the student than on subjective evaluation.' Self-selection is not a reliable basis on which to base remediation.

The conclusion which must be drawn from the above results of the analysis of the learners' scores is that neither pre-entry qualifications, nor stage or type of training, nor even self-selection is a reliable basis for deciding which learners need extra help.

TEACHING MATHEMATICS TO NURSES

Although this chapter appears in the section headed 'What to teach nurses', it is appropriate to discuss briefly here the research carried out to investigate ways in which mathematical help could be given to learners. A full report of the research can be found in Pirie (1986). In general there are three broad approaches to learning:

through class instruction, through individual tuition, or through assimilation during practical work and self-motivated use of available resources. At the time when the research was being undertaken it proved impossible to find schools of nursing prepared to put on special class teaching in mathematics for their learners. Similarly, no tutors were available to offer individual tuition in nursing mathematics. The reason for these situations was generally given as 'lack of time', although in many cases it was also due to lack of mathematical confidence among the tutors themselves. The purpose of the research was a purely practical one; to discover the most effective way, in the present training system, of offering remedial help to learners. Class teaching and individual tutorials were thus not considered to be viable options. The remaining possibilities were (1) individual tuition given by specially designed self-teaching materials, (2) individual tuition given by externally motivated use of textbooks and media, and (3) self-motivated learning on the job following a test to inform the learners of their trouble spots.

Before any comparisons could be made, the self-teaching materials had to be written and tested, since no such materials existed for British nurses. These have since been published (Pirie, 1985). A diagnostic test was also constructed to give feedback to both the learners and the research worker on the mathematical abilities of a sample of learners before and after they had received help. A detailed list of existing maths-for-nurses texts was compiled so that learners could be directed to particular materials appropriate to their needs. The test, self-help materials and book list were then used in an experiment designed to allow consideration of five questions:

(1) Will significant learning take place if learners are merely made aware of their mathematical weaknesses by means of a diagnostic test?
(2) Is either the self-teaching material or the prescribed reading list more effective than the other?
(3) Is either the self-teaching material or the reading list better than nothing?
(4) Does mathematical teaching on some topics motivate learners to learn in other topic areas?
(5) Does supervised study increase learning?

A sample of 750 students and pupils took part in the experiment, and analysis of their pre- and post-scores on the diagnostic test led to the following conclusions:

(1) Simply alerting learners to their problems by means of a test is insufficient to promote any significant learning.
(2) The self-teaching materials produced a significant increase in the number of learners achieving mastery level in every one of the topics tested.
(3) The reading list occasioned no such changes, although there was some general improvement of scores in the relevant topics.
(4) There was no 'spin-off' of learning into areas other than those specifically taught.
(5) Supervised study periods had no effect on the learning taking place.

CONCLUSION

The burden of this chapter can be summarised in three sentences. There now exists a taxonomy of nursing mathematics, and research has established that large numbers of nurses have problems with many of the topics in this list. The best form of cure is prevention, and to do this learners should be tested on entry to training for weaknesses in their mathematical abilities. They should then be made aware of their errors and offered appropriate, relevant remediation.

Responsibility for the mathematical competence of nurses must be taken seriously by tutor and learner alike. An engineer who miscalculates may waste costly materials and time; a nurse who miscalculates may kill someone.

REFERENCES

Apple, J.L. (1976) The classification of medication errors. *Supervisor Nurse, 7,* 23–25, 28–29

Ausubel, D.P. (1968) *Educational psychology: a cognitive view.* Holt Rinehart & Winston, New York

Barker, K.N. and McConnell, W.E. (1962) How to detect medication errors. *The Modern Hospital, 99,* 95–106

Cockcroft Committee (1982) *Mathematics counts.* HMSO, London

Cowan, J. (1975) The ability to appraise one's own work. *Higher Education Bulletin, 3* (2), 127–8

Daines, J.M. (1978) Self-evaluation of academic performance in a continuously assessed course of study. *Research Intelligence, 4* (1), 24–6

Gage, N.L. and Berliner, D.C. (1979) *Educational Psychology*, 2nd edn. Rand McNally, Chicago, Ill.

Huckabay, L.M.D. (1981) The effects of modularized instruction and traditional teaching techniques on cognitive learning and affective behaviours of student nurses. *Advances in Nursing Science*, 67–83

Moores, B. and Moult, A. (1979) Patterns of nurse activity. *Journal of Advanced Nursing, 4*, 137–49

Morton, J.B. and Macbeth, W.A.A.G. (1977) Correlations between staff, peer and self-assessments of 4th year students in surgery. *Medical Education, 11*, 167–70

Perlstein, P.H., Callison, C., White, M., Barnes, B. and Neil, K.E. (1979) Errors in drug computations during newborn intensive care. *American Journal of Diseases of Children, 133* (4), 376–9

Pirie, S.E.B. (1983a) *Deficiencies in basic mathematical skills among nurses*. Shell Centre for Mathematical Education, Nottingham

Pirie, S.E.B. (1983b) Nursing mathematics, in Howson, G. and Malone, R. (Eds) *Maths at work*. Heinemann, London

Pirie, S.E.B. (1985) *Maths for nursing*. Bailliere Tindall, London

Pirie, S.E.B. (1986) *Nurses and mathematics*. Royal College of Nursing, London

Scottish Home and Health Department (1967) (North Eastern Regional Hospital Board, Work Study Department). *Scottish Health Study No. 3: Nurses' work in hospitals in the N.E. Region*

Wilkinson, P.W., Noble, T.C., Gray, G. and Spence, O. (1973) Inaccuracies in measurement of dried milk powders. *British Medical Journal, 2*, 15–17

Williams, M.A. (1977) Quantification of direct nursing care activities. *Journal of Nursing Administration, 7*, 15–18, 49–51

Williamson, K.C. and White, S.J. (1974) Pharmacology competence ensured. *Hospitals, JAHA, 48*, 95–8

4

The Ward Sister: a Continuing Learner

M.F. Stapleton

INTRODUCTION

This research was concerned with the perceived needs of certain groups of trained nurses for educational opportunities to update nursing knowledge. The focus of the study was upon those of charge-nurse grade. However, the sample was designed to obtain the views of those of nursing-officer grade also, since it was considered that nursing officers could have an influence on how opportunities for such education were made available. Two specialties of nursing were included: those working in the field of 'general' nursing and those who worked as midwives. All the midwives were registered general nurses before undertaking their specialist training. Midwives, unlike general nurses, have a mandatory requirement to attend updating educational programmes at five-year intervals, and the influence that this would have on the views expressed was considered to be of interest.

Much of the initial work of the research was concerned with a need to identify components of nursing so that there could be an understanding of what nursing is before examining what is required to maintain competence by updating knowledge.

An overview of nursing and its historical content was undertaken. This led to some understanding of how and why nursing as we identify it today came into existence. Nursing history usually identifies the care of the sick as taking place through the ages by means of charitable actions, first by religious orders and later by the philanthropic effort of citizens. Wise women offered help in rural societies but families carried out most of the care of the sick until the developments of the late nineteenth century.

Foucault (1973) considered that opportunities for nursing to develop arose from the increasingly scientific approach to medicine which required a reliable, obedient, intelligent helper. Although nursing had the opportunity to develop, the close interaction with medicine was both a stimulus and a constraint. Doctors required intelligent women to help carry out their instructions. All that doctors required could have been fulfilled by literacy alone. However, medicine was and is, by its very nature, episodic (Hyderbrand, 1973), and nursing skills included an awareness of patient states that required immediate medical intervention or, perhaps more importantly, did not require such intervention. Acquiring enough knowledge to make decisions about the need for medical care as separate from nursing care developed in the vacuum which resulted from the way in which medicine was practised. To fill this vacuum, nurses needed not only knowledge, but also professional confidence robust enough to withstand the strains of this type of decision-making. Menzies (1960) describes hospital care in these terms:

> A hospital accepts and cares for ill people who cannot be cared for in their own homes. This is the task the hospital is created to perform, its 'primary task'. The major responsibility for the performance of that primary task lies with the nursing service, which must provide continuous care for patients, day and night, all the year round. The nursing service, therefore, bears the full, immediate and concentrated impact of stresses arising from patient care.

Medical care and nursing care are clearly complementary and not competitive, but the dynamic social situation in which nursing emerged and has come to professional fruition introduced many other elements which strongly influenced nursing and its organisation. Chapman (1977a) and Staunton (1979) noted that the increased knowledge available in the biological sciences, together with the expansion of social sciences, created an environment of social change which generates different expectations among people. This has its effect on what patients expect from health care and from nurses as part of health-care services.

The development of nursing from its nineteenth-century base has been fraught with difficulties and influenced by doctors who have always reacted strongly both for and against changes. The rapidity of the spread of modern nursing gives adequate testimony of the need for its development and the support of some sectors of the medical establishment of the times. However, South (1857) responded to early warnings of coming change when he wrote in defence of the existing nursing services at St. Thomas's in much the same terms that doctors of a later generation wrote about the changes that emerged from the reorganisation of nursing which followed the Salmon Report in 1966 (Dewar, 1978; Rogers, 1978).

The social changes that were occurring gave the embryonic nursing service access to the 'gentlewomen' needed by Miss Nightingale to provide educated women to spread the gospel of high standards of care of the sick (Seymour, 1956). These women moved as matrons into hospitals throughout Britain and beyond. There was also opportunity for what Williams (1978) and Dingwall and McIntosh (1978) relate to the religiosity of Victorian England, to legitimise the emergence of nursing as a respectable occupation for women.

The very existence of nursing necessitated both change and development within the occupation. Interaction between society in general and nursing, also between medicine and nursing, resulted in changes in attitudes which pushed for greater recognition by means of registration for trained nurses. Political influence was needed for this, and from 1904 until 1914 bills were brought before Parliament year after year and were rejected. There were indeed tremendous divisions within nursing as to the value of registration, some teaching hospital matrons carrying on Miss Nightingale's opposition to such a development. Miss Lüches of the London Hospital regarded such a move as degrading to nursing. In contrast Mrs Bedford Fenwick, previously matron of St. Bartholomew's, was politically very active in promoting registration (Hector, 1973). It was, however, more general political realities which, following the enfranchisement of women after the First World War, brought about registration. There was still little tranquillity in the progress of nursing in this country since the prospect of registration threatened the existence of many of the small nurse training schools across the country, and it was 1923 before the General Nursing Council produced their format for examination, and basic nurse training achieved national standards. There was not at this time, nor has there yet developed, a national standard for continuing education for nurses. The need to maintain competence by the updating of nursing knowledge has been largely unplanned and unsystematic. There has been little incentive to nurses to pursue such updating since there is no national standard in such matters. Present developments towards limited registration may well change this in the future. Evidence of educational updating may be required of registered nurses.

The literature search undertaken suggested that nursing had indeed developed a body of knowledge and that this arose from a unique mix derived from the biological and social sciences (Hockey, 1982). It also indicates that nursing exists in a dynamic social situation both within the National Health Service and in society in general. Pressures upon nursing from organisational change within the health service have resulted in a shift of emphasis from the clinical aspects of the charge-nurse role to the managerial aspects. Williams (1969) noted that managers (administrators) ignored the patient-centred elements of the charge-nurse role which the nurses themselves regarded as crucial. This emphasis on management in nursing has developed since the restructuring of nursing management following the Salmon Report (1966). It has provided a plethora of training programmes designed to reinforce and expand the management elements of the ward-sister role. These programmes were funded by Regional Health Authorities and were, in the main, the only formal programmes available to nurses which could easily be achieved. The programmes varied in quantity and quality, and few nurses attended programmes other than those offered by Regional Health Authorities, although the two to three weeks available offered no credible academic qualification. This lack of academic credibility applied equally to programmes provided for nursing officers and charge nurses. Bagley (1974) suggested that nurse managers required a similar management training to that available for membership of the Institute of Health Service Administrators. For this to happen, nurses themselves must feel motivated to demand this standard. This is unlikely to happen if employing authorities make no requirement for this when making appointments to management posts in nursing.

Berg (1973) found that nurses in the United States needed to associate continuing learning with promotion possibilities and acknowledgement by seniors, although a need for professional knowledge was also a motivating factor.

The lack of systematic updating in nursing has been noted by Auld (1979) who said that nurses continued to educate themselves only by a process of osmosis. The need for updating has been noted by Darmastaater (1977), Chapman (1977b) and Goldiac (1977). The need is based on the increasing development of the knowledge base from both behavioural and biological sciences and from the increasing expectations of people who require nursing care. There is a cost involved in both updating and retraining. Bilodeau (1969) notes the but indicates that the costs of not updating may be greater. The health of the population, like the education of the population, is a priority of national policy because deficiencies here can affect the military, technological and economic potential of the country, and nursing contributes to the nation's health both in caring for the sick and in helping to develop health programmes.

The present developments in the organisation of the health service may change the emphasis in care delivery still further in the direction of management skills.

THE DESIGN OF THE STUDY

This study examined nurses' views. Having established a framework for the activity recognised as nursing, the aim was to elicit information from nurses in the grades and specialties already identified. A survey approach was undertaken, a questionnaire being the main tool used. Two scales were developed: Scale 1 related to satisfaction with reading facilities, and Scale 2 to satisfaction with the availability of educational programmes. The questionnaire consisted of 23 questions, some dichotomous, some open-ended. Question 19 consisted of two parts, and offered four-point scales within which to answer. No appropriate tool for measuring nurse satisfaction on this topic was identified from the literature, so the questionnaire that was developed was closely examined to test its ability to measure what it was supposed to be measuring (validity). Two approaches were made. Two experienced nurse researchers were consulted during the construction of the questionnaire. A final version was presented to a group of trained nurses who had recently commenced a course of further education at a polytechnic. To elicit the information needed to meet the objectives of the research, 75% agreement on the value of the questions was required. This tested face validity only, but the limitations of this approach were accepted.

The scales that were developed to identify nurses' satisfaction were also tested to see if they were capable of producing the same results when repeated. In using the test and retest approach, correlation coefficients of 0.92 and 0.9 respectively were achieved with a 2-week interval between tests. Brown (1958) describes this as producing a coefficient of stability, and this level of reliability of the test was accepted.

Since ordinal scaling has been selected as the means of measurement, it is important to discuss the advantages and disadvantages of

this. Such scales allow views to be expressed in an order of commitment — in this case, from 'very dissatisfied' to 'very satisfied'.
Imposing numerical values upon this accepts that only those who
score in the extremes of the scale can be discriminated. In this case,
the scores were strongly skewed, which allowed the high proportion
of those scoring in the dissatisfied area of the scale to be compared
with those scoring in the 'very satisfied' area (scores of 25 or less
and scores over 75). Moser and Kalton (1972) say of such scales that
they risk 'central tendency response', but if this is not a problem,
they are a useful approach to measurement since they are easy to
understand and use. It was in recognition of the weakness inherent
in this type of scale that care was taken not to overestimate their
sensitivity.

A 10% subsample was interviewed, using a semi-structured
approach with a checklist of questions and the questionnaire as the
scene setter. The questionnaire was developed by pre-testing in
hospitals outside the sample area, and the complete questionnaire
and interviewing procedure was piloted in two stages, the second
stage testing the final version of the tools. The interviews were
designed to allow attitudes to be examined in greater depth, and
asked about the effect of organisational changes on career prospects,
and sought some information on the opportunities for systematic
updating. The respondents' views on how continuing education was
viewed by their own hierarchy was discussed to determine whether
or not they felt that such activity was encouraged, taken for granted,
treated with indifference or discouraged.

SOME FINDINGS

Satisfaction with programmes

The sample, using a cluster sampling technique, finally consisted of
284 nurses from six health authorities in one region. This was
stratified to obtain the appropriate proportion from each district,
grade and specialty. The sample was also stratified to obtain the
correct proportion from large and small hospitals. For the purposes
of the study, 'large hospital' was defined as 200 beds or more and
284 respondents represented a 75% response rate. Of the respondents 15% were male, which was close to the national proportion of
males in nursing (16%). The proportion of males among nursing
officers was higher — 21%. The distributions of respondents by

Table 4.1: Distributions of respondents by specialty and by length of time qualified

Frequency by type of nursing	
Medical/surgical	117 (41%)
Geriatric area	47 (16%)
*Specialty area	77 (27%)
Midwifery	43 (15%)
	284

Frequency by length of time qualified	
Less than 5 years	35 (12%)
5 but less than 15 years	92 (32%)
15 but less than 25 years	87 (31%)
25 or more years	70 (25%)
	284

*Includes operating theatres and outpatient departments

specialty and by length of time qualified were as indicated in Table 4.1. Of the respondents 53% were married, 11% were divorced or widowed, and 36% were unmarried. Overall, 45% had dependants: 55% of married respondents and 26% of those who were unmarried. Of those respondents who were on night duty, 63% had dependants.

Information on social status was acquired only to identify if particular groups had special problems. In fact in the analysis (stepwise regression analysis) the variable that had most influence on the levels of satisfaction with updating programmes was the presence of dependants.

Other influences on satisfaction with the availability of continuing education for nurses were

(a) Grade: Only 17% of nursing officers scored in the dissatisfaction level of the level, whereas for charge nurses the percentage was 49%. Specialty also had an influence because the proportion of general charge nurses who scored as dissatisfied was 54% and of midwifery charge nurses 19% (near to the nursing officer level).

(b) Marital status: 59% of married respondents but 37% of those who were not married scored as dissatisfied.

(c) Night duty: 59% of respondents on night duty recorded dissatisfaction.

It was interesting to discover the proportion of respondents who had attended clinical and professional educational programmes since finishing basic training. Fifty-eight per cent of all respondents had attended some clinical programme. This was reduced to 32% for those working in geriatric areas.

The above refers to attendance at programmes provided by the Joint Board of Clinical Nursing Studies, and those programmes leading to registration on any part of the nursing register.

Information relating nurses' views on the need for updating nursing knowledge and the opportunity to update showed that 94% of respondents felt some need to update nursing knowledge, but only 14% felt that the opportunity to do this was adequate. Interestingly, those qualified for less than five years reported a higher percentage of respondents in the 'great need' category (37% compared with the overall figure of 20%). Only 9% of this group saw their opportunity as being adequate.

There was a very strong impression to be gained from this research that trained nurses were conscious of a need to increase knowledge to maintain competence and were attempting to do this in a variety of ways. The most frequently mentioned of these was: journal reading — 95% of respondents referred to this; consultants' rounds — 54% of nurses; and district study episodes — 24%. In addition, 39% referred to a mixture of updating methods, which were categorised as 'own resources'; 33% of midwives saw the Royal College of Midwives as a source of updating; but only 4% of general nurses referred to the Royal College of Nursing in this way.

The types of educational programme recorded were classified into three categories for the purposes of the research. Category 1 referred to those on national registers; Category 2 mainly covered the Joint Board of Clinical Nursing Studies courses, but some other similar programmes were included; and Category 3 referred to short courses (of two to three days). In areas where there was a lower proportion of nurses who had attended formal post-basic educational programmes — for example in geriatric units — and in small hospitals, a higher percentage attended Category 2 programmes. The completed questionnaire contained a comment that indicated that this type of programme (conference, etc.) could be chosen by the participant and attended in her or his own time.

This kind of statement was confirmed during interviews in which many of those interviewed from small hospitals or geriatric units were sceptical that any funding body would consider it worth while to invest money in educational programmes for nurses in such areas.

Indeed there was a very healthy awareness among all charge nurses interviewed that money would be spent on management programmes and on programmes to prepare nurses for teaching. Programmes to sharpen the skills of those nurses who wished to remain in charge of wards and maintain clinical competence were recognised by these nurses as hard to come by. A number of nurses at interview considered that such nurses were unlikely to manage any formal programme unless they both took time out and were self-financing. Interestingly enough, these views were confirmed in Edinburgh, Manchester and Leeds, where higher education programmes in universities and a polytechnic found that nurses taking clinical options were either from overseas or were financing themselves.

Those nurses who had attended clinical courses provided by the Joint Board of Clinical Nursing Studies reported high levels of satisfaction with the programmes (all of them specialist training) in which they had participated, but many commented that, for example, earlier training in intensive therapy units could rapidly become outdated. The Joint Board of Clinical Nursing Studies was aware of these problems, but their remit did not cover continuing education. The present development of the national boards may allow some improvements here.

Satisfaction with reading facilities

In identifying libraries as a source of nursing information, it was apparent that nurses were not enthusiastic users of libraries. Some comments suggested that the lack of opportunity to use libraries, often sited near or within schools of nursing, influenced this since many (50%) worked in small hospitals (less than 200 beds) which were often some distance from these facilities. It was found in this study, as in others (Berg, 1973; Bergman, 1979) that nurses who had participated in post-basic educational programmes were more likely to use libraries than others. Among those who scored in the 'satisfied' region of this scale, 70% were participants in post-basic educational courses. Participants of such programmes were also more likely to have read a nursing journal in the week before the study and to have bought a nursing journal. Also this group of respondents was more likely to have read a medical journal in the three months before the research. Some nurses indicated their dissatisfaction with library facilities within hospitals by using the services of public libraries for professional purposes. Several reasons were given, among them convenience of opening times, and the helpfulness of the personnel. Some of these views were discussed in greater depth during interviews.

RESPONDENTS' COMMENTS

Content analysis of comments made by respondents produced further evidence that some nurses recognised that they were missing out on such opportunities to update knowledge. It is also fair to state that, from their replies, some nurses regarded libraries as repositories for textbooks rather than sources of up-to-date nursing knowledge. These were unstructured comments, freely offered. Other comments related to the need for flexible approaches encompassing the new education technologies and to a need for local publicity on the opportunities available.

Both in interview and in final comments there was reference to lack of encouragement towards continuing education: 11% of respondents wrote of this. At interview ($n = 31$), 26% felt actively discouraged. These were included within the 75% who knew that there was no money or no programme available. Indeed, at interview it was stated by a number of nurses that any kind of educational programme was seen as a kind of reward rather than as a commitment to professional competence.

Other comments that illustrated widely held views were that nurses who took time and trouble went unacknowledged, and that those who made no effort were regarded as being as competent as those who systematically did try to keep up to date. This finding was recognised in America (Berg, 1973) and Israel (Bergman, 1979).

One of the open-ended questions asked: 'Could you list any subjects which you consider could usefully be studied by nurses in charge of wards or departments to help them develop and maintain the skills required of them?' The most frequently identified need noted was for general clinical updating (25% of respondents). More than twice as large a proportion of general nurses as midwives identified this. Another category identified as a subject was 'interpersonal skills'. Twenty-two per cent of respondents referred to this. Interestingly, only 12% felt that they required updating in teaching skills. Many nurses who did not consider that they required any such updating considered that their nurse training had equipped them to teach other nurses, and some mentioned learning such skills from role models (including doctors who, one respondent noted, were teaching all the time). Marson (1979) noted that trained nurses frequently stated that 'teaching', which they identified as a didactic activity, was not part of their skills. Lelean (1973) also explained some of this reluctance when she noted the multiplicity of interruptions sustained by charge nurses, suggesting that didactic teaching in these circumstances is unrealistic. Marson (1979) writes of nurse training that it assumes that nurses learn as they work and also that nurses teach as they work. Fretwell (1980) tested this assumption in her study and found that some trained nurses did teach. She identified the key factor in the ward as a teaching environment as the charge nurse. It is she or he who controls this aspect of ward experience but the skills needed to enable this are rather sparsely catered for in both basic and post-basic training of nurses. As has been stated previously, nurses in this study did comment that specialist training was more likely to be considered if nurses were interested in a formal teaching role than if they wished to enhance skills needed at ward level.

Management training was available to nurses as an opportunity for post-basic education much more freely than was clinical updating. Seventy-five per cent of respondents had attended a management course. These programmes were available locally, in the main, funded by Regional Health Authorities, and lasted two to three weeks at most. A few nurses had also attended two- to three-day specialist management modules on topics such as law, report writing, and information presentation. As noted previously, no respondent had attended a university or polytechnic programme. Fewer nurses working part time or on night duty had undertaken management training (approximately 62% as compared with 75%).

Of those who attended such programmes 52% considered that their needs were met. Differences by grade and specialty were considerable: 91% of nursing officers in the general field, but only one nursing officer working as a midwife felt this. Twenty-seven per cent only of midwives of charge-nurse grade felt that the course met their needs. In commenting on management training, many respondents, who had not felt that they had gained sufficiently in management, felt that as a first experience of an educational programme since their basic training they had gained other advantages. Some mentioned their appreciation of the educational approach to adult learners, and the opportunity and time to meet and talk to other nurses and people in other disciplines. Also, some respondents identified that they were stimulated into rethinking some traditional practices. Many nurses also commented that the medium of industry or commerce, through which management principles and practice were identified, was inappropriate in the short programmes available to them. Most respondents identified management programmes as being: locally available and as encouraging to them as people, suggesting that such an approach to other professional updating programmes would be worth undertaking. The absence of any programmes locally which allowed systematic updating for trained nurses was commented upon; although there was both appreciation and knowledge of the Joint Board of Clinical Nursing Studies programmes available, it was recognised that these contributed to the acquisition of specialist skills and did not fulfil a need for the nurse as a continuing learner in respect of competence in the general medical and surgical wards.

Regarding the practical application of the teaching in management programmes, 57% of those who had attended such courses felt that what they were taught was not transferable to their workplace. Eight respondents in all were highly critical of all aspects of management training programmes and commented on political indoctrination, factory-based activities and total absence of reference to patients as people.

In attempting to measure nurses' satisfaction, this research approached data collecting from a number of angles:

(1) structured questions;
(2) opportunity to make undirected comments;
(3) interviews to allow more in-depth exploration of the topic.

The analysis also allowed several approaches. Using the Statistical Package for the Social Scientist (SPPS) programme, relationships were identified based on the variables of grade, discipline, span of work, shift, and hospital size, among others. Those variables showing statistically significant differences were further analysed to identify which variable was exerting the greatest influence on the scores obtained. In Scale 1 (relating to reading matter) there was little enlightenment from this, only a total of 17% of the variance being accounted for with only 7% relating to one topic — the availability of nursing journals in the workplace. In Scale 2 (educational updating programmes) 21% of variance was accounted for and, of that, 17% could be attributed to the presence of dependants.

Content analysis of final comments allowed these views also to be given weight. It was hoped that these approaches would make best use of the data offered and enable the best representation of respondents' views.

In examining nurses' perceived need for professional updating, some persistent themes emerged. Nurses recognised that they had such a need and knew that they were deficient in opportunities to increase nursing knowledge by means of reading widely since library opportunities were limited in availability. Also, nurses did not regard the use of libraries as a legitimate right. They were only slowly becoming aware of the development of district library facilities for trained staff, in the main accepting postgraduate libraries (now district libraries) as a medical domain.

A need for locally available programmes to allow systematic updating for all to be undertaken to enable the nurse to fulfil her or his own and others' expectations of the role was recognised, and there was an awareness of a need for greater flexibility in the type of educational programme offered. A need for recognition of the education undertaken may indicate the need for an 'educational unit' to emerge that is capable of incorporating different types and different forms of programme by giving different values to these as contributions to such a unit. In future, limited registration may require such evidence. However, nurses in this study indicate that there is a personal need to be able to quantify some of the varied educational inputs from which they have benefited.

At the time that the data for this research were collected, only Edinburgh, Manchester and Leeds offered an opportunity for nurses to pursue further studies as clinical nurses, and, as has been stated, few nurses who did not fund themselves could take advantage of these clinical options. Since then, programmes to extend the educational qualification of registered nurses to degree level have proliferated and many more opportunities for higher degree work in health-care studies have emerged. Where such opportunities exist within reasonable travelling distance, nurses have been quick to seek places. In this study 'reasonable' was an adjective used frequently in connection with travel, personal effort and commitment. There are therefore strong indications that those who contributed to this research were not unrepresentative of the views of their peers.

REFERENCES

Auld, M. (1979) Nursing in a changing society. *Journal of Advanced Nursing, 4*, 287–98

Bagley, C. (1974) Nursing the Salmon way. *Health and Social Service*

Journal, 84 (4374), 359–60

Berg, H. (1973) *Participant and non-participant nurses in continuing education*, DEd Thesis, Columbia University

Bergman, R. (1979) Role selection and preparation of unit head nurses. Report to Tel Aviv University of Sackler School of Medicine, School of Continuing Medical Education, Department of Nursing

Bilodeau, C. (1969) *Acquisition of skills*. Academic Press, London

Brown, A.F. (1958) *Research in nursing*. W.B. Saunders, Philadelphia, PA

Chapman, C. (1977a) *Sociology for nurses* (Nurses Aids Series). Bailliere Tindall, London

Chapman, C. (1977b) Image of the nurse. Paper presented at International Council of Nurses, 16th Quadrennial Congress, Tokyo, Japan (3 June)

Darmastaater, J. (1977) Mandatory continuing education for re-licensing. *Journal of Nursing Care, 10* (3), 26

Dewar, H.A. (1978) The hospital nurse after Salmon and Briggs. *Journal of the Royal Society of Medicine, 71* (6), 399–405

Dingwall, R. and McIntosh, J. (1978) *Readings in the sociology of nursing. Introduction, 1*. Churchill Livingstone, Edinburgh

Foucault, M. (1973) *The birth of the clinic* (translated from the French by A.A. Sheridan Smith). Tavistock, London

Fretwell, J. (1980) *Enquiry into the ward learning environment*, unpublished PhD Thesis, University of Warwick

Goldiac, K. (1977) Continuing education a 'must' for maintaining competence. Paper presented at International Council of Nurses, 16th Quadrennial Congress, Tokyo, Japan (30 May)

Hector, W. (1973) *Mrs Bedford Fenwick and the rise of professional nursing*. Royal College of Nursing, London

Hockey, L. (1982) Some methodological issues in nursing research, in S. Redfern, A. Sisson and P. Walsh (eds) *Issues in nursing research*, papers from the 22nd Annual Conference of the RCN Nursing Research Society. Macmillan, London

Hyderbrand, W. (1973) *Hospital bureaucracy*, Dunellan Publishing, USA

Lelean, S. (1973) *Ready for report nurse?* Royal College of Nursing, London

Marson, S.N. (1979) *Creating a climate for learning*. National Health Service Learning Resources Unit, Sheffield Polytechnic

Menzies, I. (1960) A case study in the functioning of social systems as a defence against anxiety. *Human Relations, 13*, 95–121

Moser, C.A. and Kalton, G. (1972) *Survey methods in social investigation*. Heinemann, London

Rogers, A. (1978) Today's nurses. *Nursing Mirror, 146* (2), 7

Salmon, B. (Chairman) (1966) *Report of the Committee on Senior Nursing Staff Structure*. Ministry of Health, Scottish Home and Health Department. HMSO, London

Seymer, L.R. (1956) *A general history of nursing*. Faber & Faber, London

South, J.F. (1857) *Factors relating to hospital nurses* (pamphlet). London

Staunton, M. (1979) New dimensions of professional responsibility. *International Nursing Review, 26* (3), 84–5

Williams, D. (1969) The administrative contribution of the nursing sister. *Public Administration*, *47* (3), 307–25

Williams, K. (1978) Ideologies of nursing, in R. Dingwall and R. McIntosh (Eds) *Readings in the Sociology of Nursing*. Churchill Livingstone, Edinburgh

5

Teaching Nurses to Teach

P. McGinnis

INTRODUCTION

Nursing is advancing in its utilisation of nursing theory and conceptual frameworks for practice, and there is evidence of such approaches underpinning practice. It would appear that before long it will be possible to describe and define 'nursing' within a professional framework. A consequence of these developments will be the need to prepare nurses in a way that will allow future nurse practitioners to be capable of meeting the health-care requirements of a modern society. What is clear is that the future holds certain changes that nurses must address. Already consumers of health care demand more, in that a disease orientation to care is less and less acceptable to them. Health is no longer seen as an absence of disease, as it was defined in the mid-1960s, but now attracts a holistic definition with a greater emphasis on the improvement of care by such strategies as patient teaching, health education/maintenance and prevention. The literature on nursing models confirms the breadth that nursing can assume when describing interventions. Orem (1980) is one such nurse theorist who describes nursing interventions towards self-care as wholly compensatory, partially compensatory, and supportive/educative. She identifies the nurse as an educator in a very broad sense, yet the provision of training for this role is scattered. There is therefore some validity in the suggestion that the arrangements for the initial and continued education of nurses are to meet today's health-care requirements.

A ROLE FOR THE EDUCATION OF NURSES

Clearly one way of expressing the objective for nurse education could be that of producing someone who can practise professional nursing. McFarlane (1977) captures this when stating: 'nursing is a practice discipline and the primary objective of education, in the profession, is education for practice'.

The position that education holds in any profession appears to be based on clearly defined goals, with a curriculum able to describe scope, content, methods and evaluation within educational practices. However, as indicated earlier, nursing is still developing, the end clearly is not in sight, and the theories and conceptual frameworks for nursing show a divergence of thinking, which creates difficulties in establishing the needs of nurses for training. However, whatever path nursing takes, a clear commitment to the following three areas is called for, namely: the practice of nursing; the teaching of nursing; and research into nursing (Nayer, 1980).

Nurses are beginning to respond to changing health-care demands and as such are reshaping the form that nursing practice will take. Some changes are in evidence within the formal curriculum for nurse training. For example, the 1982 syllabus for Registered Mental Nurses identifies a biopsychosocial input to care and goes further by expressing a unique viewpoint on the style of teaching by emphasising the role of experiential learning. Transitions are occurring as developments emerge, yet gaps can be identified between the education process and service provision (McFarlane, 1980). A greater and closer link between education and service provision is supported by the literature, one area in particular being 'joint appointees' (Esther and Bryant, 1977; Royal Commission on the National Health Service, 1979; McFarlane, 1980). The role for education could be stated as the need to increase the total number of nurses who are prepared and committed to total nursing care and who will serve as role models for others. Donovan (1971) describes the activity of education as helping, educating, and acting as a role model. The literature provokes the further questions of who should carry out the educating role and how this role should be developed in line with its involvement at all care levels, and (of particular relevance to the subject of this chapter) in line with teaching nurses to teach.

EDUCATING AND TEACHING

The role of educating and teaching can be seen as part of the same continuum. Equally, learner status to trained nurse status can be identified as progressing along a continuum. At each stage in our careers as nurses, the needs for teaching and educating change in line with role expectancy. As a learner one is receiving an education as well as teaching patients. As a trained member of staff one is receiving an education but also teaching staff and patients.

Lelean (1973) confirms this latter position when reviewing the sister's teaching role. The cumulative findings of her study of ward-sister communication suggest that a teaching role is vital at the ward-sister grade, but Lelean also makes the comment that this role remains unfilled. Is a reason for such an outcome related to the lack of theory and practice afforded to sisters in order that they can teach? Harrison, Saunders and Sims (1977) confirm Lelean's findings and suggest that we 'should not underestimate the ward sister's ability to influence the students' education. She can not only modify the students' behaviour in the ward, but influences her whole attitude to the value of the educational process.' Further evidence is available in the work of Alexander (1983), who suggests that the majority of ward staff consider that, in a situation where no clinical teacher was available, they held the responsibility for teaching students in the ward. Although teaching is accepted in the role of trained staff at ward level, Alexander spells out two serious implications of such actions, namely:

(1) Ward teaching may end up unplanned and *ad hoc* with little relevance to the total curriculum.
(2) The future of nurse teachers is questioned: will they want to join a ward team where such roles already exist, and are occupied by ward staff?

What is clear from the work of Alexander is that the ward is a very fertile arena for learning and that active experiential learning has immense potential at ward level. The ward is also postulated as the appropriate training situation by Pembrey (1980), but she identifies the role model as being the teaching agent rather than a formal teaching style. At another level Wong (1979) argues that the role of nursing training, both basic and post-basic, should cover teaching and learning more thoroughly. Wong suggests further that it seems pointless having a block on teaching or a similar topic outside of the area in which this should take place, as teaching such a topic in a school setting would create transfer-of-knowledge problems. Again this argues for the experiential value of the individual settings in which activity will take place. Research from the area of continuing education offers a further view confirming the teaching role that trained staff have. Sims, Long and Saunders (1977) reported on a study of the trained nurse in England and Wales. Questionnaires, supplemented by interviewing a subsample of respondents, identified the following continuing education needs:

(1) learning how to teach;
(2) knowing about one's own role;
(3) communication skills;
(4) clinical updating;
(5) selection/appraisal interviewing;
(6) learning to assess student nurses.

A study carried out by Stapleton (1983) six years later addressed continuing education needs within one Health Region. Her study population was the ward-sister grade and above, who were given questionnaires to complete. Interestingly three major educational needs were identified, these being

(1) interpersonal skills development;
(2) teaching skills development;
(3) clinical updating (discussed further in Chapter 4).

As a by-product of a study by Runciman (1983), sisters in the study from Scotland suggested that they needed help with teaching skills, staff appraisal and staff development. In the three studies quoted here there are a sufficient number of findings in common to direct and plan the continued education of nurses. The main finding of concern to us in this chapter is the identified need to learn and acquire teaching skills.

The role of a trained nurse clearly includes a commitment and responsibility to teaching, as already established. However, the total implications of a teaching component within a trained nurse's responsibilities are much broader when addressing the area of patient teaching.

PATIENT TEACHING AND THE NURSE

There is a wealth of literature confirming the role of the nurse in patient teaching. In midwifery and health visiting the value of teaching has been established (Chamberlain and Chave, 1977). Further confirmation is available from the work of Cima (1980) and Adair *et al.* (1980), both of which studies indicate that the scope for teaching in families with children at risk is immense. The teaching of schoolchildren in a health education setting has been shown to be effective (Biener, 1975; Addy, 1977), and at the opposite end of the age range a teaching role with the elderly has been identified. Within acute medical care there are numerous examples of the effectiveness of a teaching plan as part of total patient care. Redman (1976) outlines a total approach to patient teaching at both the individual and family levels. Group teaching of patients preparing for surgery has been evaluated (Mezzanotte, 1970) and shown to be effective, as has teaching the coronary patient (Howard and Erlanger, 1983). In all aspects of nursing, patient teaching can make an immense contribution to care. Marks (1983) examines the role of teaching with diabetic patients, and Batehup (1983) extols the values of teaching by making a link with an improvement in the stroke patient. General nursing, midwifery and health visiting utilise and report the value of teaching within caring, and clearly confirm that nursing consists of a large teaching component, but psychiatric nursing offers great scope for development.

The nurse's role in psychiatry can be seen as one of teaching patients and families and facilitating change via a teaching process. Obviously this calls for a very broad understanding of the term 'teaching', but surely that is what the education versus training debate has actually done, namely to have expanded the remit and definition of teaching.

Miller (1983) recognises and identifies this breadth of teaching involvement in psychiatry. She points out ten items on her questionnaire that revealed a teaching focus. These covered the following: role model; social skills; communication; assertiveness; behaviour therapy; daily living skills; family education; medication counselling; knowledge of the disorder; and hobbies and leisure time pursuits. Miller's work questions the simplistic definition of teaching, namely the imparting of information from one person to another, and suggests that it is a complex activity involving interpersonal skills and person-to-person behaviours.

TEACHING AND THE NURSE

Teaching as part of the nurse's role can be seen as a major issue facing nursing today. This is not a new problem, for it has been recognised for some time, but it is a significant problem that must be addressed in any future projections for the development of nursing. Any curriculum designed for nursing, whether basic or post-basic, must represent the present realities of the world of nursing and be congruent with future demands for care. Any approach must enhance the continuum of a teaching role by encompassing the teaching of learners to teach and the teaching of trained staff to teach. Clearly the link between teaching and caring has to be advanced, and for nurses this means understanding that the caring aspect of nursing has to include a greater emphasis on teaching. This can be achieved through a better assessment and planning of the care of patients. This leaves us asking the questions of how we teach nurses to teach, and what we teach them in order to fulfil this role. No single theory can account for all teaching and learning, so no single application of theory can be assumed as right for nursing. Teaching nurses to teach offers a challenge to nursing, in that a broad range of activities that facilitate the learning of teaching skills are available. Teaching a patient to self-administer insulin may well require teaching skills and strategies that align with a behaviourist approach, whereas the teaching of attitude formation to students in a ward setting in some instances may call for a more humanistic approach.

TEACHING NURSES TO TEACH

From the outset, teaching nurses to teach should be equated with education rather than training. This opinion is supported to some extent by Macmillan (1980), who offers some differentiation between education and training in the following way. She equates education with a 'whole person approach': thus the responsibility is on the learner to think and question for himself or herself, whereas training is seen by Macmillan as essentially a task-oriented process lacking the embracing concept of the 'whole person'.

This maps out our way forward quite well, namely by adding teaching to a 'whole person approach' to nursing care already in existence, the nursing process. This takes education well away from the medical-model era and its links with work and task, resulting in learning associated with procedures, to a nursing-model approach exemplified by thinking, questioning, reasoning and debate.

Greaves (1984) agrees with this approach in designing any curriculum for nursing. He postulates the dual use of existing models, namely the nursing process and the curriculum process. He goes further to confirm his intentions to 'inter-relate the central paradigms of each of these models to produce a nursing curriculum model from which nursing courses can be rationally planned, implemented and evaluated'. Greaves offers further clarification of this by stressing that:

> nurses assess patients and plan their care and evaluate this care through the nursing process and in doing so create nursing interventions or nursing events. Teachers assess their students, plan teaching, implement teaching and learning interventions, and in doing so create 'instructional events', which are evaluated for effectiveness.

It seems so obvious that these two processes interrelate and therefore would offer a natural model to follow when considering teaching nurses to teach. The nurse during an assessment of a patient defines nursing problems. Between this and the planning stage, teaching strategies may be under consideration among others. For example the assessment of a diabetic patient may include problems associated with monitoring glucose levels and administration of insulin. Part of the care plan may include teaching the patient self-administration of medication and the self-testing of urine. The nurse's role during the implementation stage would be to teach the patient accordingly using an appropriate teaching method. Clearly this teaching role suggests a need for the nurse to learn teaching skills in order to provide competent and professional care. This need creates an objective within the curriculum which in turn requires statements relating to the content, methods and evaluation. Each stage of the curriculum process can be related to each stage in the nursing process, thereby linking and integrating, at all times, skills and knowledge that can be applied to care. The use of the interrelated model, or nursing curriculum model as Greaves calls it, would allow us to identify clearly what should be taught and the emphasis required. It would be very wrong to identify teaching as a key nursing role and deal with it as a totally separate entity divorced from care when in fact the only reason for the teaching role in the first place is the demand for care made by patients. In linking the two processes so as to provide objectives related to the teaching role, it must be understood that such objectives that set out to meet the teaching role of nurses are widely generalisable and are capable of broad application over a wide range of problems presenting along the health/illness continuum. In many respects the learning objectives of a particular nursing activity should prompt broad teaching objectives. For example, if a learning objective was 'the assessment of anxiety in patients' then the objective might read:

(1) the learner will be able to identify the type and presentation of anxiety;
(2) the learner will be able to identify the degree of anxiety, the reason for its onset, the duration and the precipitating factors;
(3) the learner will be able to specify aggravating factors associated with anxiety and factors that reduce anxiety;
(4) the learner will be able to identify changes in behaviour presented by the patient as a response to anxiety.

From this set of objectives it is clear that the planning of care for the anxious patient may present with the following options:

(1) provide relief of anxiety by a biochemical intervention;
(2) alteration of intensity of anxiety by listening and understanding;
(3) use of relaxation in controlling anxiety;
(4) use of coping strategies in reducing anxiety.

From this plan it could be stated that a teaching objective exists, namely the teaching of skills or interventions based on 1 to 4 above. For example, the use of relaxation could be taught to the patient. The nurse would need a certain knowledge and skills base with which to accomplish this. Clearly teaching objectives could be identified and aimed at the learner when they arise as part of care. This does not leave out the opportunity to see teaching skills as separate and deal with them as a specific learning need. However, we are all aware of the difficulties that are apparent between teaching a skill in one area and then expecting the transfer of skills into the practice setting. A little caution is advocated here so that learning takes place in the most effective place possible.

The question raised now is what sort of skills should be defined as teaching skills and how these should be taught to nurses.

TEACHING SKILLS — WHAT ARE THEY?

There are widely held views in the literature on the education of nurses indicating that current training programmes are failing to provide learners with the knowledge and skills they require to become competent practitioners within a modern health-care system (Bendall, 1976). Two points are worth raising, namely are they not being taught specific skills related to care, or is the teaching not efficient enough to provide a base for practice? It is possible that teachers do not know what is actually needed, especially in the area of teaching skills as they relate to giving care. As one can see from studies quoted earlier, ward sisters and staff nurses argue that they need teaching skills. Has this deficit come about as a result of a lack of such inputs during student days, or do we blame post-basic continuing education?

Some of the skills needed to teach effectively can be gleaned from the work on learning environments (Leach and Lewin, 1981; Orton, 1981; Fretwell, 1982; Ogier, 1982; Marson, 1984). These research findings address the characteristics that were beneficial to learning by learners. Collectively the responses confirm the value of the social and interaction skills shown by trained staff towards learners and acclaim them specifically as being productive in meeting their learning objectives. The picture now becomes complicated to some extent. On one hand learners are spelling out exactly what they need from ward staff and the skills that meet their needs best, and on the other we have trained staff giving evidence of their continuing education needs when they describe the need for interpersonal, communication and teaching skills (Sims *et al.*, 1977; Stapleton, 1983). Clarke (1985) makes a bold statement when she confirms that good communication skills are basic to the development of teaching skills. She also advocates the role of social skills in the repertoire of skills that the teacher will need. In addition, like Harrison *et al.* (1977) she stresses the importance of the role model, and, from findings in other reports, notes that good role models for patient care are seen by learners as good teacher models. This seems to suggest that very similar skills are needed whether operating within a patient-care mode or in an educative mode. This seems to give further support for Greaves and his interrelated nursing curriculum model, in that an improvement in nursing skills may lead to the acquisition of and improvement in teaching skills. Hence the two things go hand in hand, and therefore one should not exist without the other.

Further support for the interpersonal skills approach in teaching nurses to teach is available from the general education literature on effective teaching. Teacher characteristics have been studied in great detail, and Rosenshine and Furst (1973) have written a useful review of these research studies. They have identified five consistent teacher characteristics associated with gains in pupil achievement. The works of Flanders (1970), Ryan (1960) and Berliner and Tickenoff (1976) show surprising consistency between their findings and those of Rosenshine and Furst. What is clear from these findings is that effective teachers are warm and show understanding, are organised and businesslike, and are stimulating and imaginative.

Effective teachers ask more questions and take note of pupils' feelings while acknowledging their ideas by the use of encouragement and praise. This sounds very close to the attributes one would want to see in a good nurse. In addition to the interpersonal emphasis, Smith (1971) defines teacher effectiveness as those behaviours that bring about intended learning outcomes. This is obviously a move away from the process of actually teaching into the area of measurement of outcomes. Smith has suggested that a teacher should be prepared in four areas of knowledge, namely:

(1) command of theory relating to learning and human behaviour;
(2) broad utilisation of attitudes that aim to foster learning and facilitate human relationships;
(3) command of knowledge in the relevant subject;
(4) attributes relating to technical skills of teaching that facilitate learning;

It is interesting to note that many of the factors again emphasise the area of human relationships, supported of course by technical skills in teaching.

So if nurses are to be taught these skills, which will enable them to be effective teachers, how should we address this process?

ACQUISITION OF TEACHING SKILLS

Teaching skills are not acquired without study and practice. Three stages are advocated for teaching nurses teaching skills. The first is a cognitive stage leading to the ability to form a concept of the teaching skill and its purpose. The second stage is that of practice and the realisation that teaching is a complex skill which cannot be purely learned in a classroom setting. It requires a great deal of practice to acquire a repertoire of teaching skills flexible enough to be used in a variety of combinations aimed at a variety of settings. The use of training techniques such as microteaching (Allen and Ryan, 1969) allows learners to practise teaching skills under controlled conditions. This may mean a short practice period of, say, 5 to 10 minutes with a small class of pupils and with practice of a single skill (Perrott, 1977). This approach seems ideal for the practising of such skills in a ward setting and merits further consideration by teachers of nursing.

The third stage warranting inclusion here is that of feedback and evaluation. People undergoing such practice have been shown to make substantial improvement when receiving feedback regarding performance. This need has been repeatedly demonstrated in the research studies quoted earlier. The use of microteaching would facilitate the use of video feedback and allow the teacher to take a more supervisory role within the teaching process. This fits in well with adult learners and their special needs as indicated by Rogers (1969). In view of what has been said about facilitation and supervision it would seem that the role and style that a teacher adopts have important implications for the learner.

STYLES AND ROLES FOR TEACHERS

The place of teaching within a nurse's role has been considered and confirmed as an important component. However, there is a wide range of settings for which such teaching is required. It may take place in a one-to-one setting or in a family group setting. It may focus upon a group of patients or upon a group of staff, both learners or trained. This makes the approach to teaching nurses to teach more significant. Earlier it was noted that no single application of learning theory can be assumed as right for nursing, and equally it can be assumed that no particular style or role adopted by a teacher can be right for nursing. The emphasis on relationships and climates required for effective teaching focuses our attention away from a traditional teaching role towards a supervision/counselling role or a facilitating role. The role of teacher as advocated by Rogers (1969) and confirmed by Ausubel (1975) and Maslow (1975) is a facilitator of learning. The emphasis here would be on a person creating climates, moods and relationships that allow learners freedom should they wish it, or dependence and direction should they need them. This role will enable the learner, who could be a ward sister or a student nurse, to reveal his or her true feelings and accept requirements for change. It presupposes that the role of learner is to take on and accept new demands and create actions to meet such changes. Again this process is analogous to the nursing process and fits well with Ausubel's views on meaningful learning. Ausubel suggests that the most important single factor influencing learning is what the learner already knows. Ascertain this and teach accordingly is the message. Such a facilitator role would seek to do exactly that, and leave the nurse able to meet the teaching demands based in care by creating solutions to these needs by means of a teaching framework. However, it must be noted that such a role as facilitator does have its difficulties. A major problem brought to our attention by Boydell (1976) is the difficulty learners have in defining their own needs. Boydell acknowledges this when suggesting that most learners arrive expecting all the characteristics of a traditional approach to learning. There is an understandable risk here, however. The traditional teacher role is not applicable in most nursing settings and thus a role model exemplified by a teacher exhibiting traditional values would be totally counterproductive. With the close links between teaching and care already established, the nurse must be in a position to be able to optimise every caring situation to its full. This may mean moving and shifting emphasis while interacting with the person. Accordingly flexible humanistic-based strategies are going to be far more useful and fulfilling.

In the 1982 syllabus for the Registered Mental Nurse, a unique and bold statement can be identified. This attempted to emphasise the role of experiential learning directed towards the acquisition of skills in psychiatric nursing. Surely teaching nurses to teach should take this form. Teaching nurses to teach is about communication, and Burnard (1984) focuses our attention on learning to communicate by raising the importance of talking, listening, questioning and discussing. Interestingly these are echoing the same important factors as were noted earlier in respect to the effective teacher. Burnard suggests that these factors are central to nursing functions by identifying their place in meetings, ward teaching, patient's treatment sessions, etc. He makes the point that it is not sufficient to offer nurses a few sessions on a topic and just hope that they get on with it, so it would seem that just putting on a few teaching-skills days for staff is not the answer at all.

Burnard suggests three stages in the development of interpersonal skills. Stage one is an 'unaware stage', when nurses are neither aware of the possible range of interpersonal skills nor do they notice their own behaviour. This stage is one of exploration, revelation and development of broad understanding. Stage two is the 'aware stage' where practice is encouraged and skills start taking form. Burnard reminds us that this may be a difficult time for the nurse and one that is punctuated by discomfort. This is an ideal stage to integrate microteaching techniques with supervised practice, combining teaching and caring at the grassroots. This stage should consider the nurse's attitudes, attributes and previous skill attainment in order to be motivating, stimulating and effective.

The final stage is the 'skilled stage', when the new skills, for example those concerned with teaching, are incorporated into the nurse's repertoire of behaviours. A nurse would now have teaching skills set in a human relations framework underpinned by a humanistic approach to human behaviour ready to take on demands as they occur.

To apply such skills to a work environment that has as its primary function care, certain conditions must be available. Collaboration and communication between teachers, ward staff, and learners is indicated in order to reach the fertile area in which to operate both as a teacher and as a learner. The teacher role may gain from a decentralisation away from schools of nursing into care areas. However, the blurring of roles will be a problem: namely, who does the teaching? Obviously we have to move away from this possessive behaviour and to have as our only goal an improvement in the care being given to patients. If facilitating is to be carried out satisfactorily, if teaching skills are to be introduced, and if teaching is going to be interrelated to the nursing process, then co-operation, tolerance and action are required.

A FUTURE FOR NURSING

The future of nursing is in our hands, and nursing is ready to accept change. The teaching role of staff will need addressing within a nursing framework that is conterminous with an educational framework. However, the teaching of nurses to teach should be allowed to move into an outcome-based task but should be valued for the 'process', not just the outcome. The words of Chinn and Jacobs (1978) are worthy of note when they caution that the process of developing theory and not a specific outcome should be emphasised, and that this process has greater value than the product.

Although they were addressing the philosophical underpinnings of theory development, Chinn and Jacobs' message is generalisable to our topic. Teaching and the attainment of appropriate skills need to be seen and valued by nurses as part and parcel of any care system developed. Clearly one way forward, and one with which this author agrees, is the development of nursing models for practice as these will enable us to have a common basis from which to practice, whether we are teachers of nurses or nurses working in care areas. This system would raise problems for the nurse who would look for solutions. In doing so, deficits in skills, knowledge and attitudes would be open for identification. Deficits will demand attention via educational strategies if care is to be competently addressed. Let us not take care out of teaching or teaching out of care, as this would be disastrous. A simple way to meet a learning need may be cost effective but will it be truly effective? Will it make good role models for the future? Will teaching care plans soon be evident alongside normal care plans, indicating the clear commitment to teaching? This seems yet another challenge, to see if we can integrate theory with practice, that is the theory of learning and teaching with nursing practice.

REFERENCES

Adair, D., Charlton, A., Flood, M., Harris, E., May, K., Reader, L., Robson, A. and Thompson, J. (1980) A project on home accidents. *Health Visitor, 53* (5), 158–60

Addy, M. (1977) Effectiveness of methods of teaching dental health to 9- to 10-year-olds. *Dental and Oral Epidemiology, 5,* 191–5

Alexander, M. (1983) *Learning to nurse, integrating theory and practice.* Churchill Livingstone, Edinburgh

Allen, D.W. and Ryan, K. (1969) *Microteaching.* Addison Wesley, Reading, Mass.

Ausubel, D.P. (1975) Cognitive structure and transfer, in D.J. Hounsell and N.J. Entwhistle (eds) *How students learn.* Institute for Research and Development in Post-compulsory Education, University of Lancaster

Batehup, L. (1983) How teaching can help the stroke patient's recovery, in J. Wilson-Barnett (ed.), *Patient teaching, recent advances in nursing, 6.* Churchill Livingstone, Edinburgh

Bendall, E. (1976) Learning for reality. *Journal of Advanced Nursing, 1,* 3–9

Berliner, D.C. and Tickenoff, W.J. (1976) The California beginning teacher evaluation study: overview of the ethnographic study. *Journal of Teacher Education, 27,* 24–30

Biener, K.J. (1975) Influence on health education on the use of tobacco and alcohol in adolescence, *Preventive Medicine, 4,* 252–7

Boydell, T. (1976) *Experiential learning.* Department of Adult Education, University of Manchester, p. 52

Burnard, P. (1984) A critical review of the concept of experiential learning with special reference to the training of student psychiatric nurses, unpublished MSc dissertation, University of Surrey, Guildford

Burnard, P. (1985) Learning to communicate. *Nursing Mirror, 161* (8), 30–1

Chamberlain, G. and Chave, S. (1977) Antenatal education. *Community Health, 9,* 11–16

Chinn, P.L. and Jacobs, M.K. (1978) A model for theory development in nursing. *Advances in Nursing Science, 1,* 1–11

Cima, P. (1980) Teaching parents with high risk infants in the home. *Patient Counselling and Health Education, 2* (2), 84–6

Clarke, M. (1985) The use of research reports in planning continuing education for trained nurses. *Journal of Advanced Nursing, 10,* 475–82

Dodd, A.P. (1974) Towards an understanding of nursing, unpublished PhD thesis, University of London

Donovan, H.J. (1971) Is the delivery of health care the crucial problem in nursing service? *Journal of Nursing Administration,* March/April

Entwhistle, N. and Hounsell, D. (1975) How students learn: implications for teaching in higher education, in N. Entwhistle and D. Hounsell (eds) *How students learn.* Institute for Research and Development in Post-compulsory Education, University of Lancaster

Esther, A.C. and Bryant, R.J. (1977) Educating the learners to work on the ward. *Nursing Times, 73* (2), 47

Ferguson, A.C. (1976) De-schooling nurses. *Nursing Times, 72,* 1864

Flanders, N.A. (1970) *Analysing teaching behaviour.* Addison-Wesley, Reading, Mass.

Fretwell, J.E. (1982) *Ward teaching and learning.* Royal College of Nursing, London

Greaves, F. (1984) *Nurse education and the curriculum: a curricular model.* Croom Helm, London

Harrison, J., Saunders, M.E. and Sims, A. (1977) Integrating theory and practice in modular schemes for basic nurse education. *Journal of Advanced Nursing, 2* (5), 503–19

Henderson, V. (1966) *The nature of nursing.* Macmillan, New York

Howard, J.A. and Erlanger, H. (1983) Teaching methods for coronary patients, in J. Wilson-Barnett (ed.) *Patient teaching, recent advances in nursing 6.* Churchill Livingstone, Edinburgh

Leach, J. and Lewin, D.C. (1981) *The clinical learning project: a study of factors influencing the clinical learning of student nurses.* NERU, Chelsea College, London

Lelean, S.R. (1973) *Ready for report nurse? A study of nursing communication in hospital wards.* Royal College of Nursing, London

McFarlane, J.K. (1977) Developing a theory of nursing: the relations of theory to practice, education and research. *Journal of Advanced Nursing, 2,* 261–70

McFarlane, J. (1980) *Essays on nursing.* Kings Fund, London

Macmillan, P. (1980) Paid to think? *Nursing Times, 75,* 1864

Marks, C. (1983) Teaching the diabetic patient, in J. Wilson-Barnett (ed.) *Patient teaching, recent advances in nursing 6*. Churchill Livingstone, Edinburgh

Marson, S. (1984) Developing the teacher role of the ward sister. *Nursing Education Today, 4,* 13–16

Maslow, A.H. (1975) Goals and implications of humanistic education, in N.J. Entwhistle and D.J. Hounsell (eds) *How students learn*. Institute for Research and Education, University of Lancaster

Mezzanotte, E.J. (1970) Group instruction in preparation for surgery. *American Journal of Nursing, 70,* 89–91

Miller, G. (1983) Teaching psychiatric patients, in J. Wilson-Barnett (ed.) *Patient teaching, recent advances in nursing 6*, Churchill Livingstone, Edinburgh

Nayer, D.D. (1980) Unification. *American Journal of Nursing, 80* (6), 110

Ogier, M.E. (1982) *An ideal sister*, Royal College of Nursing, London

Orem, D.E. (1980) *Nursing: concepts of practice*, 2nd edn. McGraw-Hill, New York

Orton, H. (1981) *Ward learning climate*. Royal College of Nursing, London

Pembrey, S. (1980) *The ward sister, key to nursing*. Royal College of Nursing, London

Perrott, E. (1977) *Microteaching in higher education. Research and development and practice* (monograph). Society for Research into Higher Education, University of Surrey, Guildford

Redman, B.K. (1976) *The process of patient teaching in nursing* (3rd edn). C.V. Mosby, St. Louis, MO

Rogers, C. (1969) *Freedom to learn*, Merrill, Columbus, Ohio

Rosenshine, B. and Furst, N. (1973) The use of direct observation to study teaching, in R.M. Travers (ed.) *Second handbook of research on teaching*, Rand McNally, Chicago, Ill.

Royal Commission on the National Health Service (1979) *Report*, HMSO, London

Runciman, P.J. (1983) *Ward sister at work*. Churchill Livingstone, Edinburgh

Ryan, D. (1960) *Characteristics of teachers*. American Council on Education, Washington DC

Sims, A., Long, P. and Saunders, M. (1977) *The trained nurse in England and Wales*. Research Report for the DHSS and GNC. HMSO, London

Smith, B.O. (1971) *Research in teacher education: a symposium*. Prentice-Hall, New York

Stapleton, M.E. (1983) *Ward sisters — another perspective*. Royal College of Nursing, London

Wong, J. (1979) The inability to transfer classroom learning to clinical nursing practice: a learning problem and its remedial plan. *Journal of Advanced Nursing, 4* (2), 161–8

6

Teaching Psychiatric Nursing: Interpersonal Skills

W. Reynolds and D. Cormack

In this chapter we will consider a number of distinct, although related, aspects of teaching psychiatric nursing. First, the nature of psychiatric nursing and its relationship to nursing generally will be outlined. Secondly, the use of a number of psychiatric nursing strategies will be considered: relationship therapy, counselling and psychotherapy. Thirdly, theory-based approaches to psychiatric nursing will be presented, including the application of theory to practice. Finally, one aspect of psychiatric nurse education (teaching/learning interpersonal skills) will be discussed. This section will focus on one particular aspect of interpersonal skills use, empathy.

THE NATURE OF PSYCHIATRIC NURSING

Any discussion of the education of the psychiatric nurse must be placed within the context of the *role* of the psychiatric nurse. Additionally, the role of the psychiatric nurse requires to be considered in the context of nursing generally. In some countries, such as those within the United Kingdom, psychiatric nursing is a distinct and in many ways separate part of nursing. In other countries, such as the United States of America, the generalist form of training is designed to produce nurses who will be capable of looking after a range of patient groups, including psychiatric patients. Whether or not psychiatric nursing is a distinct and separate specialty, or part of nursing generally, is by no means resolved. Henderson and Nite (1978), in that often quoted statement which seeks to define the nature of nursing, make no real distinction between psychiatric, medical, surgical or other forms of nursing. They defined the unique role of the nurse as being:

> To help people, sick or well, in the performance of those
> activities contributing to health or its recovery (or to a peaceful
> death) that they would perform unaided if they had the necessary
> strength, will or knowledge. It is likewise the function of nurses
> to help people gain independence as rapidly as possible. (p. 34)

In our view, this definition of nursing applies equally to a patient
who is recovering from an appendectomy, to a depressed person, to
an individual suffering from schizophrenia, and to an elderly person
with a broken neck of femur. Such a view is supported by a comment
attributed by Johnston (1978) to Lydia Hall (founder and director of
the Loeb Medical Center, New York) who wrote: 'Unification,
rather than fractionalisation of nursing care, is the distinctive mark
of quality nursing which can hasten recovery and rehabilitation . . .'
(p. 140).

An alternative view of psychiatric nursing is that it is fundamentally different, and distinct from, other forms of nursing. Powell
(1982) undertook a study which was designed to gain some
understanding of how psychiatric nursing students viewed their
preparation and training and, in particular, the way in which they
saw them as contributing to the prescribed role of forming relationships with patients. Powell (1982) concluded that the overall picture
was one of a limited appreciation of psychiatric nursing as being 'not
just another specialty' but as being 'the other half of nursing'. He
concluded that the role of the psychiatric nurse is quite different
from that of the general nurse, and that there is no real similarity
between the two, except that both types of nurses are responsible for
the care of patients. Powell (1982) goes on to suggest that 'The care
that the psychiatric patient requires is fundamentally different from
that required by a patient with a physical illness. The systems of care
that have developed and evolved are *not* the same' (p. 85). It is
significant that Powell justifies his assertion that the care required
by psychiatric patients is fundamentally different from that required
by physically ill persons by observing that the *systems of care* which
have developed in relation to the two types of nursing are different.

Undoubtedly, psychiatric nursing *is* different from other forms of
nursing in that psychiatric nursing involves the delivery of nursing
care to a patient population who are suffering from mental illness.
In common with all patient groups, the mentally ill person has a
range of physical needs which demand a physical nursing input.

Although, as a group, the psychiatric patient population will have more non-physical problems than the physically ill patient population, the psychiatric nurse will have to be competent in both areas of care.

The role of the psychiatric nurse has at least three major components. The first component is *custodial care* which involves the provision of the means by which the individual will physically survive. Such care involves food, fluids, warmth, clothing, a safe physical environment, exercise and the means by which physical health in general is maintained. This form of care, which is frequently undervalued by nurses and mistakenly referred to as 'basic' nursing care, is often provided by nurses while functioning relatively independently of other staff groups.

A second component of the psychiatric nurse's role is that relating to working in *support of other staff groups*. In this area, the nurse will facilitate the work of other staff groups by, for example, implementing their prescriptions, or by encouraging the patient to accept the care which other members of the health-care team wish the patient to have. For example, the nurse will administer the prescriptions of medical and paramedical staff, and occasionally has to persuade the patient to accept these. Another example of such collaboration is in the area of medical and paramedical evaluation and subsequent diagnosis, where the skills of psychiatric nurses, and their knowledge of psychiatric illnesses, are used to collect data which are subsequently passed to other staff and used as a means of diagnosing, treating and monitoring patients from a medical and paramedical viewpoint.

A third component of the psychiatric nurse's role relates to the manner in which the nurse *personally influences the mental health status of the patient*, the counselling or psychotherapeutic approach. This area of care frequently involves the psychiatric nurse in the use of one or more of a number of models of intervention, the most commonly used examples being the behavioural, psychotherapeutic and sociotherapeutic models. American writers such as Peplau (1960, 1962), Kalkman (1967) and Wilson and Kneisl (1983) are uncompromising in their view that the primary focus of psychiatric nursing should be on the counselling or psychotherapeutic role. Peplau (1962) described the psychiatric nurse as a clinical specialist in interpersonal techniques, and Kalkman (1967) referred to the nurse–patient relationship as being the basis for relationship therapy. During an extensive review of the one-to-one nurse–patient relationship, Wilson and Kneisl (1983) described an activity which parallels the principles, phases and processes of counselling and psychotherapy. These writers made it clear that they considered the nurse–patient relationship to be a form of psychotherapy, which formed the 'cornerstone' of all care delivered.

In contrast to the North American literature, writers in the UK have tended to emphasise the multi-dimensional role of the nurse. Such authors include James (1972), Altschul (1980) and Cormack (1976, 1983), who suggest that numerous other roles such as administrator, clerk and domestic help may be more important than the American literature suggests. Cormack (1985) has expressed the view that psychiatric nursing should be viewed, like all nursing, as a holistic activity, and stresses that psychiatric nursing has three major components; (i) the delivery of physical care; (ii) that which facilitates the work of other professionals; and (iii) the use of interpersonal skills by the nurse to achieve (i) and (ii) and to personally influence the non-physical health status of patients.

Research-based studies have indicated that the greatest area of difficulty in the UK lies in the use of interpersonal skills to influence the non-physical health of patients. All studies suggest that, with few exceptions, the conscious use of interpersonal skills as a nursing theory is *not* a consistent feature of psychiatric nursing. The recent major studies of psychiatric nursing undoubtedly indicate a serious discrepancy between the extent to which nurses *should* utilise interpersonal psychotherapeutic skills and the extent to which they actually *do* use these. This discrepancy has been a major feature of a number of studies carried out during the past decade (see Altschul, 1972; Towell, 1975; Cormack, 1976; and MacIlwaine, 1980). Each of these authors made some attempt to explain the discrepancy between the desired and actual use of interpersonal psycho-therapeutic skills. A major theme of the arguments presented by all authors was the extent to which psychiatric nurse training programmes failed to prepare students to utilise these skills. Altschul (1972) suggests that there is room for improvement in training to increase the nurses' therapeutic role and make them more aware of it. With the present level of skill and knowledge it would appear that (special) relationships between nurses and patients were irrelevant to psychiatric treatment.

More recent studies, including that by Faulkner (1985), suggest that there is little doubt from research findings that nurses in both hospital and community settings have serious difficulties in the structured utilisation of interpersonal skills as part of a therapeutic process. Faulkner goes on to suggest that some of these deficiencies may be due to deficits in the curricula of both basic and post-basic courses, and to a reluctance or inability on the part of tutors to use experiential methods of teaching. This general criticism of the inability, or unwillingness, of nurses to utilise interpersonal skills is not confined to psychiatric nursing. Macleod Clark (1983) criticises the extent to which surgical nurses fail to recognise the importance of nurse–patient communication (an essential feature of inter-personal relationship formation). Macleod Clark commented that despite the wide dissemination of research findings indicating the importance of nurst–patient communication, nurses on surgical wards spent little time talking to patients. The importance of interpersonal relationships on non-psychiatric nursing wards and the interrelatedness of communications and relationship skills were outlined by Ashworth (1980) when she suggested that the four main aims of nurse–patient communications were:

(1) to develop a relationship in which patients perceived the nurse as being friendly, competent, reliable and helpful, and as appre-ciating the patients' individuality and worth;
(2) to establish patients' needs as seen by them;
(3) to provide information which can be used by patients to struc-ture their expectations;
(4) to assist patients to use their individual resources and those made available to them.

Cormack (1985) implied that those researchers who concluded that psychiatric nurses had a poorly developed understanding of interpersonal skills use may have been incorrect in arriving at that conclusion so readily. Cormack wrote:

It has become fashionable in recent years to criticise the extent to which nurses fail to make use of interpersonal skills (this criticism has been particularly strong when made by nurses generally, and nurse researchers in particular). My view is that, rather than apply the concept, definition and criteria of inter-personal skills use which belong to non-nurses, we should make a fresh examination of those interpersonal skills which we *do* use. My prediction is that such an examination would add a new dimension to our understanding of interpersonal skills use in a health care setting (p. 113).

Cormack suggested that three types of interpersonal skills were being used by psychiatric nurses: direct goal (formal), direct goal (informal), and indirect goal. The direct goal (formal), of which the use of one-to-one psychotherapy designed to improve a patient's assertiveness is an example, is probably the least frequently used form of interpersonal skill. However, Cormack suggested that many researchers have (wrongly) concluded that the use of interpersonal skills by psychiatric nurses is minimal because they (the researchers) have found little use being made of direct goal (formal) interpersonal skills. The second type of interpersonal skill described by Cormack was the direct goal (informal) type, an example of which is the encouragement of a patient to 'help around the ward'. Here, rather more general and vague goals are set, and these may or may not be known to all of those involved including the patient. The general emphasis in direct goal (informal) use of interpersonal skills is on informality, an experiential approach and a commitment by nursing staff. The third type of interpersonal skill use described by Cormack is the indirect goal, an example of which is the preparation of a patient for medical treatment such as electro-convulsive therapy. Here, the nurse is utilising interpersonal skills as a means of facilitating the delivery of care which has been prescribed, or is actually being given, by another member of the health-care team.

Studies have indicated that several variables may interact to influence psychiatric nurses' attitudes towards their role in treatment. For example, Caine and Smail (1968) and Altschul (1972) concluded that the personality and sex of the nurse, the belief systems of those in authority, particularly in a hierarchical medical model of care, and the educational experiences of the nurse may be important factors. Cormack (1983) described several belief systems or models of care which may account for the role confusion that appears to exist among psychiatric nurses. These approaches to care include the medical, behavioural, sociotherapeutic and psycho-therapeutic models of care. Shanley (1984) expressed the view that the sociotherapeutic model offers a better framework for the psychiatric nurse to fulfil a psychotherapeutic role than does the medical model, due to its greater emphasis on interpersonal experiences and on the personal qualities of staff. Shanley's conclusion supported Towell (1975) who demonstrated that only in a therapeutic community ward was there a tendency for nurses to focus on the personal feelings and perceptions of patients.

Irrespective of the model of care, most writers imply that nurse–patient interactions have the capacity to facilitate a helping relationship between the nurse and her patient. Studies by Altschul (1972) and Cormack (1976, 1983) indicate that both nurses and patients value verbal interactions and feel that the quality of the nurse–patient relationship is an important component of care. These studies also revealed that nurses *and* patients believe that if the nurse displayed poor interpersonal skills, such as a lack of neutrality or understanding of the patient's world, relationships could be damaged. Thus, whether psychiatric nursing should focus on a counselling framework, or whether counselling skills such as empathy, warmth and geniuneness (Rogers, 1957) should be viewed as part of the psychiatric nurse's repertoire of skills, there is general agreement that the learning of interpersonal behaviours that facilitate a helping relationship is a legitimate part of psychiatric nurse education.

The implication of this for psychiatric nurse training is that teachers must identify the central interpersonal skills which facilitate a helping relationship, and identify from theories of learning how best to help students acquire therapeutic behaviours, and how to assess these. At present, the means by which teachers attempt to facilitate and assess students' interpersonal behaviours are largely unknown. A research-based study by one of the writers (WR) provides some information about how Scottish teachers teach and assess students' empathy (a core characteristic of an effective interpersonal relationship) during the progress of a psychiatric nursing module.

Differences existed between students' educational experience in three colleges of nursing in respect of where, how and when they were taught about empathy. For example, one college (A) provided intensive experiential learning in the clinical area, and another (C) provided education that was almost entirely classroom-based.

RELATIONSHIP THERAPY

Various terms have been used to describe the manner in which psychiatric nurses can personally influence the mental health of their patients. A review of the literature provides a great deal of support for the view that the traditional nurse–patient relationship, counselling and psychotherapy, are overlapping therapies (see Table 6.1). This is in spite of Cormack's (1985) view that the nurse–patient relationship is neither borrowed from, nor imposed by, other professional groups. Cormack suggests that the unique feature of this approach is that it is built into the normal, day-to-day contact

Table 6.1: A comparison of the one-to-one nurse–patient relationship and counselling/psychotherapy

One-to-one nurse–patient relationship	Counselling/psychotherapy
'Relationship therapy refers to a prolonged relationship between a nurse therapist and a patient, during which the patient can feel accepted as a person of worth, feels free to express himself without fear of rejection or censure and enables him to learn more satisfactory and productive patterns of behaviour' (Kalkman, 1967, p. 226)	'A special relationship between a patient and a psychotherapist which is aimed at helping the patient change problematic feelings, cognitions and/or behaviours' (Ruch, 1984, p. 18)
'The one-to-one relationship between psychiatric nurse and patient is a mutually defined, mutually collaborative, goal-orientated professional relationship. It may involve informal relationship work or more formal relationship work, including crisis intervention, counselling or individual psychotherapy' (Wilson and Kneisl, 1983, p. 882)	'A special relationship between a patient and a therapist, through which they mutually define problem areas and negotiate goals for the patient in an effort to increase the patient's satisfaction with living' (Wilson and Kneisl, 1983, p. 137)

between nurses and patients. While not disagreeing with Cormack's view, Reynolds (1985) has suggested that the nurse–patient relationship, counselling and psychotherapy, are all variations of a psychotherapeutic approach which depends upon the same repertoire of therapist behaviours. This is apparent when definitions of relationship therapy, counselling and psychotherapy are compared.

It can be seen from these definitions that relationship therapy and counselling, or psychotherapy, share many common features (see Table 6.2), and that nurse–patient relationship therapy is a more extensive form of relationship building in the sense that it involves more than formal therapy sessions. This would support Cormack's (1985) view that the nurse–patient relationship is unique, and Reynolds' (1985) opinion that all forms of relationship building are similar.

Table 6.2: Common features and differences between one-to-one nurse–patient relationships and counselling/psychotherapy

One-to-one nurse–patient relationship	Counselling/psychotherapy
A process of relationship building	A process of relationship building
Involves prolonged one-to-one contact over a time period	Involves prolonged one-to-one contact over a time period
Involves a specific type of verbal and non-verbal interaction	Involves a specific type of verbal and non-verbal interaction
Involves a problem-solving relationship that passes through various stages	Involves a problem-solving relationship that passes through various stages
May be informal or formal	Always formal. Requires more structure, planning and consistency

THE FACILITATIVE CONDITIONS OF RELATIONSHIP BUILDING AND DETERMINANTS OF THERAPEUTIC OUTCOME

We have said that therapeutic outcome (patient growth) within the nurse–patient relationship, or a counselling or psychotherapy relationship, is dependent upon the same therapist behaviours, irrespective of the technique used. Rogers (1957), the strongest advocate of this idea, has suggested that three essential conditions are both necessary and sufficient for patient growth. These central and core therapist behaviours have been defined as empathy, warmth and genuineness. It is argued that when patients experience high levels of these interpersonal behaviours, they learn to be non-defensive and to be able to consider alternative coping strategies (Table 6.3).

It has been argued that the nurse–patient relationship is a form of psychotherapy and that the core behaviours of empathy, warmth and genuineness are the most important determinants of therapeutic outcome. These behaviours are central to all forms of relationship building, and are more important than the therapist's technique.

The hope that traditional classroom teaching alone will facilitate nurses' psychotherapeutic skills has not been supported by the literature or by our experience. The indications are that traditional (teacher-centred) teaching has been a spectacular failure. For this reason, teachers and researchers have turned their attention towards experiential (student-centred) teaching in both the classroom and clinical situations, where close supervision has been provided (Reynolds, 1982, 1984; Reynolds and Smoyak, 1983; Reynolds and

Table 6.3: The interpersonal strategies associated with relationship building

Empathy (understanding)	Warmth (respect)	Genuineness (trust, openness)
Accurate perception of current feelings/ concerns, and communication of this understanding to the patient	Commitment by the therapist in his effort to understand. Involves spontaneous participation	Therapist is without facade or pretence. Involves being real self and non-defensive
Key behaviours: Conveying empathy	Conveying warmth	Conveying genuineness
1. Listen for the feeling behinds words	1. Focus on the here and now (immediacy)	1. 1–3 under 'Warmth' apply
2. Attend to non-verbal communication	2. Use open rather than closed questions	2. Avoid frequent interruption of silence, but sometimes use it as a focus
3. Avoid taking on the patient's feelings as if they were your own	3. Remain neutral and accept the patient's reality	3. Respond to direct questions, then re-focus on the patient
4. Reflect the patient's own feeling tone and language	4. Allow the patient to make the decisions, avoiding advice or manipulation of their thoughts	4. Be consistent and predictable
5. Convey impressions in a manner which allows the patient to refute your observation if you are wrong	5. Focus on the patient rather than yourself	5. Don't allow external stressors to alter your behaviour
	6. Seek clarification when message is unclear	

Cormack, 1985). Central to the experiential approach is Bandura's (1977) view that, in order to acquire behaviours, students must have a role model and must be provided with the opportunity to receive reinforcement during practice.

THEORY-BASED APPROACHES TO PRACTICE

Consider what a nurse might decide to do when faced with the need to respond to a given situation. Fox (1983) suggests that

> . . . she might simply try the first idea to come to mind and see if it worked. If it did not work, then she might try the second idea she thought of, and the third, until one worked sufficiently well. Or she might seek to determine what others have done before her in similar situations. Or, she might rely on directives from those in authority, or more senior to her. (p. 7)

This approach, which clearly lacks any theoretical or scientific basis, probably represents the most common approach to problem-solving in nursing today. The difficulty with this approach is that solutions are often accepted without question or rationale, and even if the nurse finds a solution, she cannot be certain that it is the best one, or that it is one that will enable the patient to achieve an optimal level of health.

A nursing theory can explain why people behave in a particular way, thus guiding the nurse to the prescription of appropriate intervention, and helping her to predict outcome. Thus, nursing becomes a structured and less haphazard activity, eliminating trial and error. Furthermore, unless the nurse has a theory, she must rely upon the biases and belief systems of physicians and others in authority to decide what the nursing role is. Whenever possible, a theory that has been tested by a rigorous research method should be selected because the scientific approach considers the available care options and establishes criteria for determining which is the best solution.

It is probable that there is not a single theory of nursing, and that nurses should borrow from several theoretical approaches to guide their actions, that is, they should adopt an eclectic approach. The first goal of the nurse educator should be to help students understand and apply existing theories of human behaviour to nursing practice. This is a prerequisite of nurse-directed practice and of the most appropriate nursing care.

The manner in which a theory can be applied to practice can be examined by considering some of the principles underlying general systems theory; the Orem self-care model; the Roy adaptation model; operant learning theory; Rogers' client-centred model; and Peplau's interpersonal model.

The application of theory to nursing practice

As is the case in much of the literature on the subject, we use the terms 'theory' and 'model' interchangeably. Although presented separately, the extent to which all models/theories overlap and inter-relate is recognised. The manner in which a theory can be utilised to guide practice can be examined by considering some principles underlying a selection of available theories and their applications to clinical practice. Some of these theories have been developed by nursing theorists, and others are borrowed from related disciplines.

General systems theory

A system may be defined as a set of related units. Systems theory (see Table 6.4) has applications to the living organism, family units or other social systems such as psychotherapeutic groups or a ward system (Von Bertalanffy, 1969). This theory is popular with family therapists, for example, where the tendency is to focus on the relationship between separate parts (family members), rather than on individual classical psychopathology. Thus general systems theory also has application to the manner in which individuals live together in an institution, and is relevant to social or milieu therapy.

Orem self-care model

In brief, the self-care model developed by Orem (1980) (see Table 6.5) guides nursing processes to help patients establish, maintain, or increase self-care and self-determination in day-to-day living. Using this approach, the nurse can thus help patients avoid a lifestyle of institutionalised psychiatric chronicity and dependency.

Roy adaptation model

A major focus of the Roy adaptation model (see Table 6.6) model is directed towards how man maintains his biopsychological integrity. The view is taken that people are constantly faced with the need to adapt to environmental stimuli (Roy, 1976). There are

133

Table 6.4: General systems theory

Principles	Possible clinical applications	Predicted outcome
There is a constant action-reaction between associated things	a) Examination of inter-related parts by means of: clinical staff meetings; one-to-one nurse–client relationships; therapeutic discussion groups; psychodrama sessions; and activity groups, e.g. creative art, creative writing	Increased staff and client awareness of each others' behaviour, feelings, thoughts Improved communication between significant others (i.e. more open, honest and insightful)
Systems may be open or closed in terms of change, challenge and new ideas	b) Attempt to improve flexibility and adaptation to change by: clinical staff meetings; individual staff counselling or career development service; therapeutic discussion groups; client–staff suggestion books; and individualised care plans	Support is experienced during stressful change Ideas are shared in a non-defensive manner Everyone contributes and feels part of the treatment plan Care is individualised
Individuals within social systems tend to compensate when balance is upset, which often results in dysfunction	c) Maintain balance (homeostasis) by providing opportunity to learn more adaptive responses to changes and threat by: clinical staff meetings; one-to-one nurse–patient relationship therapy; therapeutic discussion groups; psychodrama; diversional activity, e.g. games, ward chores, outside visits; setting therapeutic limits to behaviour	Open communication system and increased self-awareness result in less need to be preoccupied with 'covering up' Adaptive coping mechanisms learned Relief and diversion from 'here and now' problems are provided

Table 6.5: Orem self-care model

Principles	Possible clinical applications	Predicted outcome
Man is a holistic individual, i.e. a unity that can be viewed as functioning biologically and in a psychosocial manner	Individual care plans based on a problem-solving approach that encompasses all aspects of human needs	Total care is administered, which increases the potential for the client to achieve his optimal health goals
Man's functioning is linked to his environment, i.e. stressors and support networks available. Health is achieved when adequate support networks are available	Reduce stressors by helping the client to deal with stress effectively and strengthening his support networks by: one-to-one relationship therapy; therapeutic discussion groups; psychodrama; relaxation exercises; prompt administration of PRN medication; a varied daily routine suited to the client's resources; place client in situations where friendships can be facilitated, e.g. social events, holidays, etc.; facilitate links with home and friends by letter writing and home visits. Network with helping agencies to resolve issues of finance and housing	Client develops self-awareness when she/he examines stressors and effectiveness of coping strategies Client's repertoire of coping skills is increased Stressors are reduced Support networks are increased
	Client develops self-awareness when she/he examines stressors and effectiveness of coping strategies	
Nursing interaction should aim to support life processes, promote normal functioning, maintain growth, development and maturation, and prevent or control disease	Assessment of client's level of self-care Provide experiences/support networks that maximise the client's level of self-care/independence by: psychotherapeutic experiences to promote learning/trust and self-esteem; access to resources such as transport, wheelchairs, writing materials, newspapers and TV; teaching clients by helping them obtain knowledge or skill essential to a particular series of acts; assisting or doing things for the client which he is unable to do for himself, e.g. feeding, washing and dressing, etc.	These actions provide a wholly compensatory, partially compensatory or supportive educative nursing system of care Each action has as its goal establishing, maintaining or increasing self-determination in day-to-day living

Table 6.6: Roy adaptation model

Principles	Possible clinical applications	Predicted outcome
The nature of man's interaction with the internal and external environment is a response to changes in the environment	Assessment of biological functioning, e.g. rest, sleep, nutrition, elimination, etc. Assessment of client responses to environmental change (external)	Staff understand more clearly the relationship between environmental change and levels of adaptation. The client is viewed in a holistic manner
The combined effect of environmental stimuli and client's coping strategies determines man's level of adaptation, which is expressed as behaviour through: physiological functions; self-concept; role functioning; and interdependence. The nurse's role is to make interventions that help clients to achieve the most adaptive behaviour possible	Reduce environmental stressors (internal and external) by prompt administration of medication, e.g. tranquillisers, hypnotics, antacids, etc; control of external stressors by means of group support, individual relationship therapy, flexible routines, realistic demands, etc. This relates to the manipulation of the client's milieu by the nurse and could include strategies such as protecting the client from other clients who are threatening, i.e. don't sit them together at the same lunch table, etc.\nAll strategies previously discussed that build trust or promote a more effective self-concept or disrupt hallucinations, etc.	The client experiences less stress. Client's need for symptom defences are reduced, e.g. greater control is achieved over hallucinations. Client achieves a higher level of adaptation by improving his physiological function, self-concept, role functioning and interdependence

various modes of human adaptation which provide a framework on which to base psychiatric nursing practice.

MODELS OF CARE

The theories described so far are unique in the sense that they tend to prescribe an intervention which includes a broad spectrum of strategies or treatment approaches. Some theories prescribe a much narrower, or more specific, approach towards *intervention*, and, as a consequence, may be regarded by some individuals as models of care rather than eclectic theory approaches. The following fall into that category.

Operant learning theory

Operant learning theory (see Table 6.7) is a good example of an explanation system, or theory, which has become associated with a major model of care, the behaviour modification approach. It has application in the treatment of a range of symptoms, including the reversal of ineffectual and conditioned responses to the hospital environment. The operant learning theory involves the nurse providing reinforcement and taking on the role of teacher when specific responses are not included in the patient's repertoire of existing skills (Barker, 1982).

Rogers' client-centred model

This approach (see Table 6.8), based on Rogerian theories (Rogers, 1957) of the necessary and sufficient conditions for patient growth, has the potential for the use of a great deal of the communication strategies taught to the nurse. The focus is on the 'here and now', and the view is taken that the patient has the capacity to accept responsibility for making changes in his lifestyle. This model fits comfortably into the sociotherapeutic model of care, and into the psychotherapeutic model.

Interpersonal model

This approach (Peplau, 1952, 1969; see Table 6.9) borrows from the Rogerian model and the operant learning theory. It involves both a non-directive approach and the idea that the nurse is a teacher through a role-modelling function. The main emphasis is on the development of a problem-solving relationship.

Nurses require an understanding of one or more theories to guide

137

Table 6.7: Operant learning theory

Principles	Possible clinical applications	Predicted outcome
Learning occurs when a stimulus is presented. A response occurs and the response is reinforced. Stimuli can be defined as environmental events that influence a person's behaviour. Responses are discrete behaviours elicited by the stimuli. Reinforcement, either positive or negative, refers to the consequences of behaviours which are elicited by the stimuli; non-reinforcing consequences refer to punishment	Make a behavioural assessment by recording objective data which tells: what the maladaptive behaviour is; what causes/influences maladaptive behaviour; what reinforces or maintains maladaptive behaviour. When doing this it is essential to record verbal and non-verbal behaviour during interactions between client and environment Select new target behaviour and a motivator. This means determining what responses will be reinforcing for a particular client Make a behavioural contract with the client Intervention. This refers to a consistent application of an appropriate reinforcer and possibly teaching new skills (role modelling) Evaluation of the outcome during clinical staff meetings	Staff and client are able to select suitable behavioural goals together. Nursing responses/approaches are consistent. Maladaptive behaviour is weakened. Client learns more adaptive behaviour. The motivation of everyone concerned is constantly monitored

Table 6.8: Rogers' client-centred model

Principles	Possible clinical applications	Predicted outcome
A client has the ability within a non-directive counselling relationship to focus on his immediate difficulties, to validate his experiences, and to examine his strengths and coping strategies. Non-directive means the absence of manipulation of the client's thinking, and the ability to be open and empathetic	Facilitation of the client's ability to form trust relationships and to make changes in their life by provision of one-to-one counselling sessions which expose the client to the following therapist behaviours on a regular and consistent basis: cognitive empathy, neutrality, genuineness (congruence with feelings), avoidance of manipulation (non-possessive therapist warmth/unconditionality of regard), focusing on the here and now, assisting client to clarify unclear communication	The client learns to trust the therapist, i.e. feelings of threat are reduced. Client is able to 'grow' i.e. to examine more adaptive coping mechanisms

Table 6.9: Peplau's interpersonal model

Principles	Possible clinical applications	Predicted outcome
Intervention begins with the development of a relationship with the client	Individualised and primary nursing approach	Facilitates the trust relationship through various phases of orientation, testing out exploitation, and resolution
The unique focus of nursing rests in the reactions of the client to the circumstances of his illness. Therapy is directed towards helping clients to gain intellectual and interpersonal competencies beyond those they had at the point of illness. In doing this the nurse may assume any of the six identified roles: stranger, resource person, teacher, leader, surrogate, counsellor	One-to-one counselling sessions on an informal and formal basis (Rogers' approach) Therapeutic discussion groups Nurse constantly examines her own values, beliefs, attitudes and behaviours which may be reflected in speech, dress, biases, etc. Psychodrama/social skills groups with props, e.g. baking utensils, films, photographs, videos, etc. Therapeutic community concepts where significant power and control are devolved to juniors and clients Needed facts are readily provided, e.g. regarding medication, limits to behaviour, treatment goals, etc. Assistance is provided with eating, self-care, etc. as required (balanced against capability and treatment goals)	The client feels accepted as a person of worth, feels free to express himself without fear of rejection or censure, and is able to learn more satisfactory and productive patterns of behaviour. Social control is learned; gratification can be delayed. Dependency on others is reduced. Self-esteem is improved. Client's biological needs and safety are protected

their actions, otherwise they are dependent upon the subjective views of others, past practice, or trial and error to guide nursing interventions. This may result in the selection of nursing responses which are the least effective, or which are damaging to the patient's health needs. We have discussed several theoretical approaches that can be utilised to guide nursing practice, and have examined what such theory suggests nurses *can do* to help patients achieve their maximum health goals. When the nurse learns to utilise theoretical approaches, the role of the psychiatric nurse is determined by the principles underlying each theory.

The implication of this for nurse educators is that students need to be helped to relate theory to practice. Reynolds and Cormack (1985) emphasised that students often struggle to formulate operational nursing activity from a multiplicity of theories and psychiatric concepts. Students may know *what* to do, but often experience difficulty in learning *how* to do it. Reynolds (1982) suggested that *all* teachers should demonstrate nursing theory to the student, arguing that role modelling and supervised practice was the only logical answer when the student asked questions such as 'How do I motivate the patient'? or 'What do I do or say when the patient says that he feels hopeless or lonely?' Support for this view may come from a research-based investigation of students' empathy, currently being done by one of the writers (WR). Trust empathy did not significantly change between measures in any of the subject groups whereas state empathy did. This suggests that state empathy (empathic behaviour) may be a more promising target for nurse educators. This view is strengthened by the Hogan Empathy Scale and stable factors of personality on Cattell's ICPF test and the tendency for state empathy scores on the Empathy Contract Rating Scale to correlate only with factors C and Q4, which have been shown by past studies to be state factors rather than stable components of personality.

TEACHING/LEARNING INTERPERSONAL SKILLS

Although the role of the psychiatric nurse is multi-dimensional and utilises both psychomotor and interpersonal skills, the area that is now receiving the greatest amount of attention in psychiatric nursing is that concerning teaching and learning skills relating to the development of therapeutic relationships. Although learning how to develop and maintain such relationships would be helpful to *all* health professionals, and to those they care for, these skills have

141

proved to be the most difficult ones both to teach and to assess.

Aidroos (1985) suggests that it is often unclear what nurse teachers mean by interpersonal skills, and that where interpersonal skills have been defined there is often no clear indication of when or how the student is provided with an opportunity to learn and rehearse these skills. French (1982) notes that accreditation procedures tend not to consider how nursing is taught within the curriculum. Arguably, there is a need to examine what is meant by interpersonal skills, and to consider how teachers have attempted to teach and assess those attitudes and behaviours that are characteristic of an effective interpersonal relationship. In this section we focus on the acquisition of core interpersonal behaviours, namely empathy, warmth and genuineness, which Rogers (1957) described as the necessary and facilitative conditions for effective interpersonal communications and relationship building. Muldary (1983) argues that these three conditions are interrelated and interact in such a way as to increase and complement each other. For example, the communication of empathy (the ability to see things from another person's point of view) can be hollow or threatening if the emphasising individual is not without a façade and is not genuine. Irrespective of this interdependence, many theorists have suggested that empathy may be the most significant facilitator of therapeutic outcome during formal counselling interviews, or in informal psychotherapeutic interactions. La Monica *et al.* (1976) write: 'Empathy has been found to be the primary ingredient in any helping relationship' (p. 447).

A review of the literature reveals that numerous writers have suggested that what Hurst (1985) has referred to as 'progressive nurse education' may well be the most effective way of developing core interpersonal behaviours. Hurst has suggested that progressive learning is characterised by its student-centredness; the teacher's role is changed to one of facilitator, with encouragement of an open/critical approach and the emphasis on experiential learning. By contrast, Hurst describes traditional teaching as being teacher-centred, with emphasis on rote learning and on the use of didactic teaching methods. Thus, the non-traditional approach towards the teaching of interpersonal skills, irrespective of whether it occurs in the classroom or in clinical areas, relies upon a variety of student-centred experiential activities.

Several North American studies support the view that traditional didactic teaching, of itself, will not enable professionals to facilitate the 'growth' of other people. Following a review of 81 studies, Taft

(1955) reported a lack of correlation between the amount of theory taught and the ability to judge others. This point was emphasised by Chance and Meaders (1960) who explored the relationship between increased 'psychological mindedness' (knowledge of psychology) and empathy. The results demonstrated that empathy significantly decreased as psychological mindedness increased.

There is evidence in the literature of an increasing awareness of the need to educate and train care givers more effectively in interpersonal skills both in the classroom and in clinical areas. Clinton (1985) argues that *equal* attention should be given to classroom and clinical education. However, recent research stressed the ward learning environment as being the main influence on what and how students learn (Davis, 1983). Some UK writers have been uncompromising in the recognition that interpersonal qualities are best facilitated during supervised clinical practice (Reynolds, 1982, 1984, 1985; Reynolds and Cormack, 1982; Ellis and Watson, 1985).

Several classroom methods of teaching interpersonal skills have been described in the literature. These include psychodrama (Dietrich, 1978) and experiential learning in small groups, which have variously been described as human relations seminars and sensitivising training (Thompson, Lakin and Johnson, 1965; Logan, 1969) and modelling (Layton, 1979). Layton's modelling procedures are based upon research by Bandura (1977). That study suggested that much behaviour is learned from the observation of other people and the consequences of their behaviour. Bandura emphasised that, without an initial model from which to imitate and learn, the individual might well not acquire appropriate behaviours.

Evaluation of several teaching programmes has tended to consist of unstructured data obtained from students' diaries, or from formal and informal discussions with students. However, the Layton study, which examined an approach to teaching empathy, utilised the empathy subscale of the Barret–Lennard Relationship Inventory. Results indicated that teaching was effective for junior students, but was less effective for senior students. Layton concluded that it was important to introduce the learning of core conditions of the interpersonal process early in training. Some studies (Coleman and Golfka, 1969; Farrell, Haley and Magnasco, 1977) have attempted to improve research methodology by utilising control groups to make comparisons with the experimental group. Results from these studies have been promising.

Several studies have been conducted to test a method of increasing the facilitative conditions of relationship building which involves a combination of didactic and experiential methods. One such study (Carkhuff and Truax, 1965) involved the supervisor didactically teaching the trainee his accumulated clinical and research knowledge concerning therapeutic behaviours. Experiential learning was then provided which required the trainees to rate the therapist's ability during taped patient–therapist interactions. In addition, trainees role-played, and finally their initial clinical interviews with patients were taped and rated. Assessment of the facilitative conditions was measured on scales such as the Truax Accurate Empathy Scale, which, in previous extensive research, had proved to be both a reliable and valid measure. It was found that in less than 100 hours of training the trainees could be taught to function at levels of effective therapy similar to those of more experienced therapists. What was not made clear in that study was how long-lasting the effect of the treatment was.

In recent years, descriptions of structured clinical supervision programmes for psychiatric nursing students have appeared in the UK literature, and arguments have been advanced for a greater concentration of teaching resources in clinical areas. The teaching methods proposed in the UK literature closely follow the approaches used in the American system of nurse education where teachers often have a dual classroom/clinical teaching role. These teaching programmes are both student- and patient-centred (clinically focused).

Central to the patient-centred approach is the notion that the teacher should provide the therapeutic role model which Bandura (1977) argues is essential if individuals are to acquire effective therapeutic behaviours. In addition, 'raw' clinical data from student-patient verbal and non-verbal interaction is observed and/or recorded. These data are utilised during supervision sessions with teachers (clinical conferences), which are intended to facilitate the students' personal and professional development. Blake (1956) points out that students need constructive practical experiences so that they may acquire new patterns of behaviour, and that their practice must have a demonstrable relationship to theory.

The rationale for the provision of clinical supervision by nurse teachers is partly based on the assumption that, in order to teach clinical skills, the teacher must personally practice these skills. Reynolds (1985) suggested that it was unfortunate that nurse teachers in the UK had largely delegated responsibility for the supervision of students in clinical areas to practising nurses, because these nurses may not have teaching skills or the time or motivation to teach. Furthermore, clinicians may not share the teacher's perception of the nurse's role. For example, if clinicians do not view counselling skills as being a primary function of the psychiatric nurse, it is unlikely that students will observe or practise counselling unless their teacher is actually present.

A further argument advanced for the need for teachers to participate in clinical nursing practice with their students is the view that student growth is, like patient growth, dependent upon a non-threatening relationship between teacher and student. This point was made by Bregg (1958) who claimed that the interaction between teacher and student is an important influence not only on the learning experience, but also on the student's personal and professional growth.

Reynolds (1985) and Hughes (1985) described the teacher–student relationship as replicating the nurse–patient relationship in the sense that it progresses through the same phases, namely orientation, testing out, working together and termination. This view is similar to that expressed by Blake (1956) who argued that, in order to display central interpersonal behaviours such as empathy, the student must experience empathy from her teacher. This point has also been emphasised by other writers such as Von Bergen and Cline (1956) who wrote: 'In order to learn how to give help, the student needs to experience receiving help. This experience is made available to her through her relationship with the instructor' (p. 152).

Reynolds (1985) proposed that, although the trust relationship between teacher and student may begin in the classroom, it *cannot* be developed or fully utilised only in the classroom. Such development can *only* occur during prolonged clinical supervision when students experience emotionally determined attitudes which can, and often do, influence the learning process. Peplau (1957) suggested that what student nurses actually experience when patients are anxious, or express feelings of worthlessness, resentment, or hatefulness, influences these situations. Understanding by the nurse of her own behaviours can only occur when she is helped by her teacher to examine what is felt, thought and done during a type of supervision which provides security and freedom. Reynolds (1985) described the use of a student daily journal as a tool for facilitating self-awareness. Journal content was examined during clinical conferences and included an account of each day's experiences, along with a description of the student's perception of herself and

145

others. The effectiveness of clinical supervision remains a fertile area for nurse researchers.

SUMMARY

Psychiatric nursing is part of all nursing and contains a number of role elements, one of which is the therapeutic use of the nurse–patient relationship. Although there is disagreement in the literature about those aspects of the psychiatric nurse's role that make it different from other nursing specialties, all writers imply that the skills of relationship building are central to all aspects of that role. It is argued that, in order to teach and assess interpersonal skills, teachers must define what they mean. Rogers (1957) has postulated that the central characteristics of effective therapist communication are empathy, warmth and genuineness. A voluminous amount of research suggests that empathy is the major determinant of a helping relationship.

Psychiatric nurses should consider theoretical frameworks which may form a useful basis for guiding practice. Theories can suggest what nurses can do, or should do, to facilitate the maximum amount of physical *and* psychosocial health of their patients. A theory-based approach to practice will answer the question, 'What is psychiatric nursing?'

Research suggests that traditional classroom-based didactic teaching is an ineffective way of increasing students' interpersonal skills. A variety of non-traditional approaches have been adopted which combine the classroom and clinical areas. These approaches have been student-centred and focused on experiential learning. It is argued that the teacher–student relationship has the capacity to develop the student's self-awareness, and that this relationship can only be fully developed *and* exploited during supervised clinical practice. Reynolds (1982, 1985) and Reynolds and Cormack (1985) suggest that students learn to trust the teacher when they share patient-centred activities. These papers described clinical supervision programmes for student nurses during psychiatric nursing modules. The focus was upon the student's working day and patient contacts during a variety of activities which included counselling, psychotherapeutic group work, and social activities such as ball games, creative art, and visits to restaurants, shops or the theatre.

A variety of teaching tools which have been developed and described by Reynolds (1985) and Reynolds and Cormack (1985) were utilised during these teaching programmes. They included process recordings from one-to-one clinical interviews, a daily activity guide which was used to plan and assess a variety of shared problem-solving activities with patients, and a sociometric analysis of group dynamics during the progress being made by psychotherapeutic groups. An essential feature of these teaching programmes was the role-modelling function of the teacher and the use of pre- and post-clinical conferences between student and teacher, which were used to plan and evaluate care. The essential theme of Reynolds' (1982, 1984, 1985) arguments is that in order to teach psychiatric nursing effectively, the teacher *must* practice psychiatric nursing. To do otherwise is to risk 'professional suicide', in Reynolds' (1982) view, in the sense that teachers become de-skilled, and their teaching becomes irrelevant to the delivery of nursing care.

REFERENCES

Aidroos, N. (1985) Interpersonal skills: building block for a core component in nursing curriculum, in A. Altschul (ed.) *Psychiatric Nursing*. Churchill Livingstone, Edinburgh

Altschul, A.T. (1972) *Patient–nurse interaction: a study in acute psychiatric wards*. Churchill Livingstone, Edinburgh

Altschul, A.T. (1980) The role of professionals. *Nursing Times, 76*, 555–6

Ashworth, P. (1980) *Care to communicate: an investigation into problems of communications between patients and nurses in intensive therapy units*. Royal College of Nursing, London

Bandura, A. (1977) Self-efficacy: towards a unifying theory of behaviour change. *Psychological Review, 84*, 191–215

Barker, P. (1982) *Behaviour therapy nursing*. Croom Helm, London

Blake, F. (1956) The supervisor's task. *Nursing Outlook, 4*, 641–3

Bregg, E. (1958) How can we help students learn? *American Journal of Nursing, 58*, 1120–2

Caine, T. and Smail, D. (1968) Attitudes of psychiatric nurses to their role in treatment. *British Journal of Medical Psychology, 41*, 193–7

Carkhuff, R. and Truax, D. (1965) Training in counselling and psychotherapy: an evaluation of an integrated didactic and experiential approach. *Journal of Consulting Psychology, 29*, 333–6

Chance, J. and Meaders, W. (1960) Needs and interpersonal perceptions. *Perspectives of Psychiatric Care, 28*, 200–10

Clinton, M. (1985) Training psychiatric nurses: why theory into practice won't go, in A. Althschul (ed.) *Psychiatric nursing*. Churchill Livingstone, Edinburgh

Coleman, M. and Golfka, P. (1969) Effects of group therapy on self-concept of senior nursing students. *Nursing Research, 8*, 274–5

Cormack, D. (1976) *Psychiatric nursing observed; a descriptive study of the work of the charge nurse in acute admission wards of psychiatric hospitals*. Royal College of Nursing, London

Cormack, D. (1983) *Psychiatric nursing described*. Churchill Livingstone, Edinburgh

Cormack, D. (1985) The myths and realities of interpersonal skill use in nursing, in C. Kagan (ed.) *Interpersonal skills in nursing: research and applications*. Croom Helm, London

Davis, B.D. (ed.) (1983) *Research into nurse education*. Croom Helm, London

Dietrich, G. (1978) Teaching psychiatric nurses in the classroom. *Journal of Advanced Nursing, 3*, 525–34

Ellis, R. and Watson, C. (1985) Learning through the patient. *Nursing Times*, 20 February, 52–4

Farrell, M., Haley, M. and Magnasco, J. (1977) Teaching interpersonal skills. *Nursing Outlook, 25*, 322–5

Faulkner, A. (1985) The organisational context of interpersonal skills in nursing, in C. Kagan (ed.) *Interpersonal skills in nursing research and applications*. Croom Helm, London

Fox, D. (1983) *Fundamentals of research in nursing*. Appleton-Crofts, Norwalk, CT

French, S. (1982) Design for accreditation of educational programmes in nursing, in M. Steed-Hensonson (ed.) *Recent advances in nursing*. Churchill Livingstone, Edinburgh

Henderson, V. and Nite, G. (1978) *Principles and practice of nursing* (6th edn). Macmillan, London and New York

Hughes, C. (1985) Supervising clinical practice in psychological nursing. *Journal of Psychosocial Nursing, 23*, 27–32

Hurst, K. (1985) Traditional versus progressive nurse education: a review of the literature. *Nurse Education Today, 5*, 30–6

James, D. (1972) Trends in nurse education. *Nursing Times, 68*, 29–31

Johnston, C.M. (1978) Total patient care v. task allocation: a student nurse's point of view, in H.O. Allen and J. Murrell (Eds) *Nursing training: an exercise in curriculum development*. Macdonald & Evans, Plymouth

Kalkman, M. (1967) *Psychiatric nursing*. McGraw-Hill, New York

La Monica, E. (1981) Construct validity of an empathy instrument. *Research in Nursing and Health, 4*, 389–400

La Monica, E., Carew, D., Winder, A., Haase, A.M. and Blanchard, K. (1976) Empathy training as the major thrust of a staff development program. *Nursing Research, 25*, 447–51

Layton, J. (1979) The use of modelling to teach empathy to nursing students. *Research and Nursing Health, 2*, 163–76

Logan, D. (1969) Action-orientated group therapy as a training method for psychiatric student nurses. *Journal of Psychiatric Nursing and Mental Health Services, 7*, 201–6

MacIlwaine, H. (1980) The nursing of female neurotic patients in psychiatric units of general hospitals. PhD thesis, University of Manchester

Macleod Clark, J. (1983) Nurse-patient communication: an analysis of conversations from surgical wards, in J. Wilson-Barnett (ed.) *Nursing research, ten studies in patient care*. Wiley, Chichester

Muldary, T. (1983) *Interpersonal relations for health professionals: a social skills approach*. Macmillan, London and New York

Orem, D. (1980) *Nursing concepts of practice*, 2nd edn. McGraw-Hill, New York

Peplau, H. (1952) *Interpersonal relations in nursing: a conceptual frame of reference for psychodynamic nursing*. Putnam, New York

Peplau, H. (1957) What is experiential teaching? *American Journal of Nursing*, *57*, 884–6

Peplau, H. (1960) Talking with patients. *American Journal of Nursing*, *60*, 964–6

Peplau, H. (1962) Interpersonal techniques: the crux of psychiatric nursing. *American Journal of Nursing*, *62*, 50–4

Peplau, H. (1969) Theory: the professional dimensions, in M. Norris (ed.) *Proceedings of the First Nursing Theory Conference*. Department of Nurse Education, University of Kansas

Powell, D. (1982) *Learning to relate*. Royal College of Nursing, London

Reynolds, W. (1982) Patient-centred teaching: a future role for the psychiatric nurse teacher? *Journal of Advanced Nursing*, *7*, 469–75

Reynolds, W. (1984) Psychiatric nursing in the USA. *Nursing Mirror*, *158*, 25–7

Reynolds, W. (1985) Issues arising from interpersonal skills in psychiatric nurse training, in C. Kagan (ed.) *Interpersonal skills in nursing: research and applications*. Croom Helm, London

Reynolds, W. and Cormack, D. (1982) Clinical teaching. An evaluation of a problem-oriented approach to psychiatric nurse education. *Journal of Advanced Nursing*, *7*, 231–7

Reynolds, W. and Cormack, D. (1985) Clinical teaching of group dynamics: an evaluation of a trial clinical teaching programme. *Nurse Education Today*, *5*, 101–8

Reynolds, W. and Smoyak, S. (1983) Interview — Bill Reynolds. *Journal of Psychosocial Nursing*, *21*, 38–46

Rogers, C. (1957) The necessary and sufficient conditions of therapeutic personality change. *Journal of Consulting Psychology*, *21*, 95–103

Roy, C. (ed.) (1976) *Introduction to nursing: an adaptation model*. Prentice Hall, New York

Ruch, M. (1984) The multidisciplinary approach: when too many is too much. *Journal of Psychosocial Nursing*, *22*, 18–23

Shanley, E. (1984) Evaluation of mental nurses by their patients and charge nurses. PhD Thesis, University of Edinburgh

Taft, E. (1955) The ability to judge people. *Psychological Bulletins*, *52*, 23

Thompson, V.D., Lakin, M. and Johnson, B.S. (1965) Sensitivity training and nursing education. *Nursing Research*, *14*, 132–7

Towell, D. (1975) *Understanding psychiatric nursing*. Royal College of Nursing, London

Von Bergen, R. and Cline, N. (1956) Some aspects of learning how to supervise. *Nursing Outlook*, *4*, 152–4

Von Bertalanffy, L. (1969) General systems theory and psychiatry: an overview, in W. Gray, B. Duhl and N. Rizzo (eds) *General systems theory and psychiatry*. Little, Brown, Boston

Wilson, H. and Kneisl, C. (1983) *Psychiatric nursing*, 2nd edn. Addison-Wesley, San Francisco, CA

7

Teaching Psychiatric Nursing: Curriculum Development for the 1982 Syllabus

S. Sankar

INTRODUCTION

The 1982 Mental Nursing Syllabus of training for psychiatric nurses differs quite radically from the previous syllabuses, and in order to ascertain the feasibility of a smooth transition from the present syllabus (GNC, 1974) to the new syllabus (ENB, 1982), against the background of curricular activities within the school of nursing, a pilot study was undertaken with a new intake of psychiatric nursing students during their 'Introductory Course'. The programme for this intake of learners was designed on a model that reflected the new syllabus, and was essentially orientated towards the development of psychiatric nursing skills. The process of curriculum planning and development in one school of nursing is described in this study through action planning, utilising an adapted version of Bolam's (1975) conceptual framework on educational innovation. Since the 1982 Syllabus complements the notion of education and training, it lends itself to the integration of the 'process' and 'product' models to develop a curriculum model that is eclectic in nature. This has led to the development of a 'competency-based curriculum model' within the framework of a 'process' and 'product' approach for curricular activities towards implementing the 1982 Syllabus in one school of nursing. This study also gave the opportunity to test on a small scale the choice of Peplau's (1952) interpersonal model of nursing and its integration for curriculum development, in order to understand its practical implications and suitability for the enhancement of intrapersonal and interpersonal skills.

THE DRAFT SYLLABUS

A draft syllabus for Mental Nursing was issued by the General Nursing Council for England and Wales (now the English National Board) in October 1981. Copies were circulated to all interested parties and comments were sought. The draft proposed a 'skills-based' approach to curriculum design, and included four sections:

(1) nursing skills;
(2) organisation and management skills;
(3) professional skills; and
(4) the knowledge base.

With the exception of section 4, the sections included a further four subsections using the framework of a model of nursing care, the nursing process, and specific secondary skills were identified under the usual four stages of the nursing process, identified as assessment, planning, implementation and evaluation.

In October 1982, the General Nursing Council (GNC, 1982) indicated that response to the draft syllabus was a general welcome for the approach and content proposed. Following some amendments to the draft, the Council approved the 1982 Syllabus for implementation and urged schools of nursing to implement it at the earliest possible date.

THE 1982 MENTAL NURSING SYLLABUS

The 1982 Syllabus of training for Part 3 of the Professional Register is presented with several amendments to its draft format, and identifies only two sections: nursing skills, and nursing knowledge. The 'nursing skills' section incorporates the first three sections in the draft into one, and identifies the specific skills required of the psychiatric nurse by listing them as those concerned with assessment; planning; implementation; and evaluation — the four stages of the nursing process (Figure 7.1)

The 1982 Syllabus places a lot of emphasis on 'self-awareness', and this heads the list of skills under assessment. The knowledge base (Figure 7.2) is also radically shifted in the 1982 Syllabus, and greater emphasis is placed on the social and applied sciences area. This applies particularly to sociology and psychology, and includes many more areas in these disciplines not previously included in the draft syllabus.

152

Figure 7.1: Development of nursing skills in the psychiatric nurse (1982 Mental Nursing Syllabus)

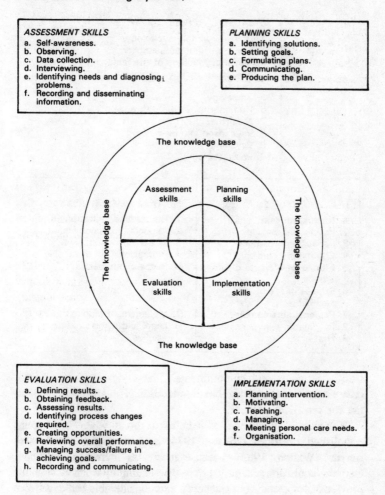

ASSESSMENT SKILLS
a. Self-awareness.
b. Observing.
c. Data collection.
d. Interviewing.
e. Identifying needs and diagnosing problems.
f. Recording and disseminating information.

PLANNING SKILLS
a. Identifying solutions.
b. Setting goals.
c. Formulating plans.
d. Communicating.
e. Producing the plan.

EVALUATION SKILLS
a. Defining results.
b. Obtaining feedback.
c. Assessing results.
d. Identifying process changes required.
e. Creating opportunities.
f. Reviewing overall performance.
g. Managing success/failure in achieving goals.
h. Recording and communicating.

IMPLEMENTATION SKILLS
a. Planning intervention.
b. Motivating.
c. Teaching.
d. Managing.
e. Meeting personal care needs.
f. Organisation.

THE PLANNING OF CURRICULUM CHANGE

The process of change

An awareness of change strategies may facilitate the consensual process through persuasion and manipulation. As an example, the normative re-educative change strategy (Bennis, Berne and Chinn, 1970) assumes that individual staff members hold a variety of

Figure 7.2: The knowledge base (1982 Mental Nursing Syllabus)

Part 1
SOCIAL AND APPLIED SCIENCES
1. Developmental psychology.
2. Studies of human sexuality.
3. Social psychology of the family and other primary groups.
4. Psychology.
5. Sociology
6. Human physiology with anatomy.
7. Medicine.
8. Psychosomatic medicine.
9. Psychiatry.
10. Pharmacology.

Part 2 *NURSING STUDIES*	*Part 3* *PROFESSIONAL STUDIES*
1. Nursing process.	1. History and philosophy.
2. Psychiatric nursing.	2. Aspects of economics.
3. Rehabilitation studies.	3. Health service studies.
4. Community studies.	4. Professionalism of nursing.
5. Studies of the care of the elderly.	5. Research studies.
6. Studies in specialised techniques.	6. Teaching studies.
7. Personal nursing care.	7. Management studies.
8. Psychiatric emergencies.	8. Legal and adminstrative studies.
9. First aid.	

values, attitudes and commitments. These views, if recognised, create an environment wherein co-operation is obtainable and potential for growth is fostered.

However, any change is seen as a threat when it threatens established practices (Nisbet, 1974) and produces a 'defensive retreat' (Walton, 1983), because it creates increased workload, anxiety, confusion, identity crisis (for example, when it de-skills previous competencies in teachers), and considerable backlash from those who firmly believe that 'things were much better as they were!'

Therefore, any change strategy that is used for developing the curriculum must be thought through very carefully, and all available resources (manpower and materials) must be utilised to the best advantage, and managed with wisdom, not fear.

Action planning

For the purpose of describing the action planning which influenced the process of curriculum development, a model developed by Bolam (1975) is set out. His model draws considerably on systems theory. Bolam states that in any innovation process we can usefully distinguish between four major factors (Figure 7.3).

Figure 7.3: Conceptual framework for the study of educational innovation. (Adapted from Bolam, 1975)

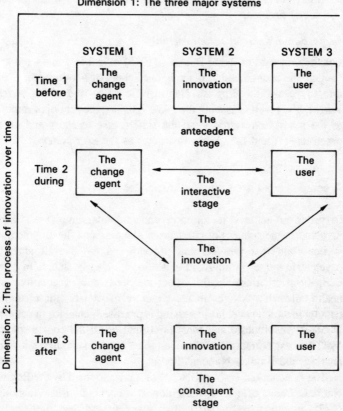

Dimension 1: The three major systems

Dimension 2: The process of innovation over time

(1) *The change agent system.* Often referred to as the change advocate, consultant or innovation. May be an individual teacher, head or adviser, a teacher centre, a local authority, a national body, or even the national government.

155

(2) *The innovation system.* Bolam (1975) distinguishes between *innovation* as being an intentional and deliberate process, and *change* which can also include accidental or unintentional movements or shifts.

(3) *The user system.* This is the system which is either inventing or adapting an innovation, or is being aimed at by a change agent.

(4) *The process of innovation over time.* This consists of three stages, namely (a) 'before' stage, (b) 'during' stage, and (c) 'after' stage. It sees the notion of innovation as a dynamic social process that takes place over a period of time during which the innovation may be redefined and modified as a result of that social process.

Using Bolam's model in our 'setting'

For the purposes of using Bolam's (1975) model to understand and manage the change taking place in one school of nursing, it is possible to regard the English National Board as the *change-agent system*, as a result of issuing the 1982 Syllabus; the school of nursing as the *innovation system*; and the staff (nurse teachers and nurse practitioners) and the clients (learners) as the *user system*.

A competency-based curriculum model

In order to achieve a common understanding among all those involved in the process of curriculum planning and development, it is important that the learning process and the overall aims of psychiatric nurse training and education be clearly stated. In addition, the curriculum should reflect the needs and expectations for health care, the changes in the structure of society, the changing context in which psychiatric nursing is practised, changes in patterns of health and illness, and most important of all the content of the 1982 Mental Nursing Syllabus compiled by the statutory body for nursing, the English National Board.

The Educational Policy (GNC, 1983) now adopted by the English National Board offers the definition of a curriculum by Stenhouse (1975) as guidance for curriculum planning and development. 'A curriculum is an attempt to communicate the essential principles and features of an educational proposal in such a form that it is open to critical scrutiny and capable of effective transition into practice.' It is not intended to make a critical review of curriculum models here, but it is worth noting that Stenhouse's definition of curriculum reflects a 'process model' that concentrates on 'planning' and the integration of theory and practice. According to Stenhouse the curriculum must be understandable and workable through the overall educational process and evaluation is viewed as a learning experience rather than measuring outcomes from pre-specified behaviour — a major problem with the process model!

Alternatively, the 'product model' advocated by, for example, Bobbit (1981), Wheeler (1967) and Tyler (1949) allows for pre-specified behaviour — 'the end product' to be evaluated by observing behaviour — and therefore is suitable in curriculum areas that emphasise information and skills development, as in the 1982 Mental Nursing Syllabus. Therefore, by using a taxonomy of educational objectives, a major contribution to the 'objective model' (see, for example, Bloom 1979; Krathwohl, Bloom and Masia, 1964; and Harrow, 1972) in the areas of cognitive, psychomotor and affective domain, it is possible to measure the pre-specified, observable behaviour.

In the light of the 1982 Mental Nursing Syllabus, which complements the notion of education and training, it seems appropriate to integrate the 'process' and 'product' models and develop a curriculum model that is eclectic in nature. This idea prompted me to develop a 'competency-based curriculum model' within the framework of a 'process' and 'product' approach (Figure 7.4). This 'model' centres on the following general objectives:

(1) to offer professional preparation that is consistent with current and projected educational needs of the psychiatric nurse, and;
(2) to provide competency in concepts and strategies related to psychiatric nursing skills in working with persons of all age groups.

The choice for an eclectic approach is consistent with:

(1) the values and beliefs held by the school of nursing;
(2) the overall educational philosophy;
(3) our choice of Peplau's interpersonal model of nursing;
(4) the 'model' also lends itself to the integration of theory and practice.

Figure 7.4: A competency-based curriculum model (1982 Mental Nursing Syllabus)

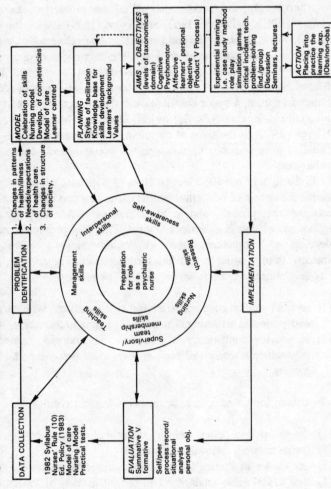

A REVIEW OF PEPLAU'S INTERPERSONAL MODEL OF NURSING

Peplau's developmental model of nursing originated from her theory of nursing — the fostering of personality development in the direction of maturity. In *Interpersonal relations in nursing* (1952, p. 16) Peplau summarises her concept of nursing as follows:

> Nursing is a significant, therapeutic, interpersonal process. It functions co-operatively with other human processes that make health possible for individuals in communities. In specific situations in which a professional health team offers health services, nurses participate in the organization of conditions that facilitate natural ongoing tendencies in human organisms. Nursing is an educative instrument, a maturing force, that aims to promote forward movement of personality in the direction of creative, constructive, productive, personal and community living.

Peplau elaborates on the definition of nursing and the role of the nurse. She defines nursing as 'a human relationship between an individual who is sick, or in need of health services, and a nurse especially educated to recognise and to respond to the need for help' (Peplau, 1952). Peplau gives two general categories that summarise interacting conditions essential for experiencing health:

(1) the physiological demands of a human organism that require material conditions manipulated on behalf of the welfare of an individual or group;
(2) interpersonal conditions that are individual and social, and that meet personality needs and allow the expression and use of capacities in a productive way.

Peplau builds her nursing theory upon two assumptions. First, 'The kind of person each nurse becomes makes a substantial difference in what each patient will learn as he is nursed throughout his experience with illness' (1952, p. 11); she emphasises personal maturity and self-awareness: 'The extent to which each nurse understands her own functioning will determine the extent to which she can come to understand the situation confronting the patient and the way he sees it' (Peplau, 1952, p. 11). The second assumption is stated as 'fostering personality development in the direction of maturity and is a function of nursing and nursing education. It

159

requires the use of principles and methods that permit and guide the process of grappling with everyday interpersonal problems or difficulties' (Peplau, 1952, p. 11). This assumption stresses the importance of the educational preparation of the nurse. The problem-solving method is seen by Peplau as the best means to achieve this end of maturation.

Peplau has identified specific roles that the nurse assumes in a nurse-patient relationship. The first role is that of a stranger. 'A stranger is an individual with whom another individual is not acquainted' (Peplau, 1952, p. 44). It may seem obvious that nurse and patient are strangers at first, but preconceived ideas of each others' role may cloud this perception. Peplau urges the showing of the usual courtesies to the 'patient-stranger' as to any other guest in any situation. This implies '(1) accepting the patient as he is, (2) treating the patient as an emotionally able stranger and relating to him on this basis until evidence shows him to be otherwise' (Peplau, 1952, p. 44).

The nurse is a resource person. The resource role is fulfilled by providing specific answers to questions usually concerning greater problems. This role involves providing knowledge as well as expertise in technical procedures. The nurse as a resource person must discern between questions that require direct, straightforward answers and those that involve feelings that require application of the principles of counselling.

Another role is that of counsellor. The counsellor is 'one who, through the use of certain skills and attitudes, aids another in recognising, facing, accepting, and resolving problems that are interfacing with another person's ability to live happily and effectively' (Nursing Theories Conference Group, 1980, p. 76).

The nurse as a teacher utilises many different methods. Peplau emphasises beginning from what the patient knows and proceeding towards what he wants to know and is able to use. She recommends learning by experience as opposed to traditional teaching methods.

The role of leadership is another nursing function. Peplau views the nurse as a democratic leader. Democratic leadership implies that everyone participates in an endeavour. The nurse, then, is the one 'who carries out the process of initiation and maintenance of group goals through interaction' (Nursing Theories Conference Group, 1980, p. 76). Peplau warns that the patient may overvalue the nurse's goals as his own and become dependent. Nurses can recognise this blind acceptance and work with the patient towards a solution to his problem.

Often nurses are cast into surrogate roles, replacing or symbolising someone else. This may come about in different ways. The behaviour of the nurse, her appearance or her attitude may remind the patient of someone else, and he may react to her, consciously or unconsciously, as if she were that other person. These feelings will shape the expectations the patient has for the nurse and form his reactions to her. Peplau emphasises that the nurse needs to be herself; the nurse can use this surrogate role as a learning experience for the patient to become more in touch with his feelings and thought processes.

Peplau identifies four sequential, overlapping and interrelated phases during the interpersonal relationship of nurse and patient: orientation, identification, exploitation and resolution. In the initial phase, orientation, the nurse and the patient come together as strangers.

In getting orientated to the nurse, the patient needs to know her name, he needs to know that she is a qualified nurse, what she may be called upon to do, the time limits which govern the duration and frequency of his contacts with her, and what she will do with the information she gets from him (Peplau, 1960, p. 965).

The orientation phase involves the nurse, patient and family in defining the problems.

The focus during the orientation period is on the needs of the patient. The needs may be psychological or physiological. The patient may or may not be aware of his needs, but his behaviour will be attempting to compensate for this deficit. Needs are not always obvious and must be clarified. The nurse may take on the role of resource person or counsellor in establishing the patient's needs.

Needs may give rise to anxiety. Decreasing anxiety is another important aspect of orientation. The nurse needs to provide information to the patient about what to expect so that he can be psychologically prepared. Peplau feels that, by naming the unknown, tension anxiety will be decreased.

The next phase is identification. During this phase the patient selectively responds to people he feels can meet his needs. Three ways in which the patient responds have been identified by Peplau: '(1) participate with and be interdependent with the nurse, (2) be autonomous and independent from the nurse, or (3) be passive and dependent on the nurse' (Nursing Theories Conference Group, 1980, p. 78). The patient may respond differently depending upon his needs, how they are being met, and his perceived control of the situation. The goal of the nurse is to facilitate forward movement of personality to displace feelings of helplessness and hopelessness with feelings of creativity, spontaneity and productivity.

The identification phase is also a time of observation for the patient and the nurse. This has two purposes: '(1) the development of clarity about the patient's preconceptions and expectations of nurses and nursing, (2) the development of clarity regarding the nurse's preconceptions and expectations of a particular patient and his skills in handling his problem' (Peplau, 1952, p. 37). Communication can clarify misconceptions and strengthen the nurse–patient relationship so that the patient can begin to deal with his problem.

Exploitation is the phase when the patient fully utilises the service available to him. As he attempts to take full advantage of health services, the patient may make more demands during recuperation than when seriously ill. Other patients are more self-directing in their use of the services. The nurse's role is to provide a non-threatening environment in order that progress can be made towards the resolution phase.

The final phase of Peplau's interpersonal process is resolution. The identified needs have been met by the efforts of both nurse and patient. Resolution is a time to dissolve the bonds of the therapeutic relationship. Peplau stresses that the patient's psychological needs may continue after the physiological needs are met. Likewise, it may be difficult for the nurse to free herself from the bond of the relationship. When resolution, a freeing process, is sequential to previous phases, the nurse and the patient become stronger, maturing individuals.

'Professional closeness' is a phrase Peplau (1969) uses to delineate an essential element of the interpersonal relationships process. The focus of the nurse should be exclusively on the interests, concerns and needs of the patient. Physical closeness is an element of this style. Empathetic linkages are another aspect of professional closeness, but unlike social interpersonal intimacies the patient is always the sole focus.

In order for the nurse to maintain professional closeness, she must be a mature individual able to utilise social situations or staff interactions to meet her own needs. During professional time, she must focus solely on patients' needs, showing 'that she can put herself aside and can bring all her capacities, talents, and competencies to bear upon the life of another person to the end that the person will grow and learn something new and in effect be strengthened in a favourable direction' (Peplau, 1969, p. 349).

PEPLAU'S MODEL — IMPLICATIONS FOR CURRICULUM DEVELOPMENT

Since the nursing curriculum is designed with an end product — 'a nurse' — as its goal, a nursing model such as Peplau's (1952) would facilitate the examination of a conceptual framework within which both these processes may occur, and shape the nurse's attitudes, values and beliefs about man, society and health. This, Stevens (1979) argues, facilitates an induction into the nursing milieu and ethos for the nurse. Stevens also argues that the choice of a single model of nursing for curriculum development enables the integration of knowledge, and helps teaching staff in the selection and organisation of learning experiences.

Peplau's model provides the framework on which interpersonal skills could be developed, and the choice of an interpersonal model fits in well with our local setting, where training/education is provided. Peplau's model also complements our design of a competency-based curriculum model. In response to our choice of Peplau's model, it became necessary to develop a conceptual framework on which components of interpersonal skills could be interlocked and developed as a process (Figure 7.5). This idea of a conceptual framework was developed by adapting the findings of a research study (Sparks, Vitalo, Cohen and Cahn, 1980) in the area of interpersonal skills.

The idea of three interlocking circles at the centre illustrating the 'student–subject–setting' components was originally developed by Chater (1975), and adapted here to demonstrate the interaction between the 'setting' — the school of nursing, the 'student' — which recognises the individual differences in learners, and 'the subject' — to allow for the integration of knowledge, skills and attitudes during the process of interpersonal skills development.

The whole of the conceptual framework then allows for the integration of Peplau's interpersonal model of nursing to dictate the 'core' content of psychiatric nursing practice, which Derdiarian (1979) advocates as a way of subscribing to the goals of nursing practice. In this context, the 1982 Mental Nursing Syllabus could be safely rationalised.

Figure 7.5: Development of interpersonal skills in the psychiatric nurse (1982 Mental Nursing Syllabus)

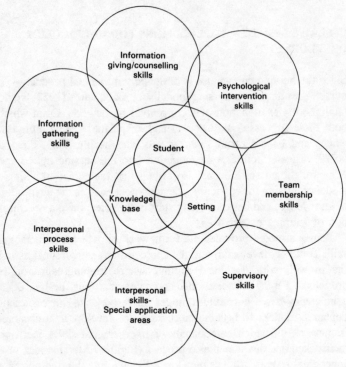

Pilot Study

The purpose of the Pilot Study was to ascertain the feasibility of a smooth transition from the present syllabus (GNC, 1974) to the new syllabus (ENB, 1982), against the background of those curricular activities, described earlier, pertaining to the 1982 Mental Nursing Syllabus.

All basic nurse training programmes begin with an 'Introductory Course'. The ENB in their training regulations (ENB 1982 — Appendix 1) stipulate that a period of 28 weeks/140 days will be organised for theoretical instruction by the school of nursing, and that it *must* start with an *introductory* period of 6 weeks' duration. This is usually followed by a period of clinical experience of approximately 10 to 12 weeks, and ends with a 'consolidation' block of 1

Figure 7.6: Integrating theory and practice. Preparation for first practical experience (pattern of 'Module' 1982 Mental Nursing Syllabus)

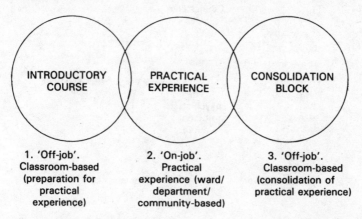

INTRODUCTORY COURSE	PRACTICAL EXPERIENCE	CONSOLIDATION BLOCK
1. 'Off-job'. Classroom-based (preparation for practical experience)	2. 'On-job'. Practical experience (ward/ department/ community-based)	3. 'Off-job'. Classroom-based (consolidation of practical experience)

or 2 weeks in the school of nursing, before repeating the cycle for other experiences (Figure 7.6). The intention for an Introductory Course of 6 weeks' duration is clearly stated in the regulations. In response to this a programme for the 6 weeks was devised, allowing for an introduction to the broad areas of the syllabus, but emphasis was placed on the development of intrapersonal and interpersonal skills (Figure 7.7), supported with the appropriate subjects from the knowledge base.

The learners spent approximately 25 hours a week during the Introductory Course, and out of this about 5 hours a week were spent on the wards — 'on-job' activities gaining practical experience with the support and supervision of nurse teachers. The emphasis during these placements was on the enhancement of psychiatric nursing skills through the application of the appropriate knowledge base required from 'off-job' (classroom-based) activities. The remaining 20 hours of the week's programme were devoted to introducing the broad areas of the syllabus, and a proportion of this time was allocated to self-directed learning activities.

Since the emphasis in the Introductory Course is on the introduction of psychiatric nursing skills, it seemed appropriate to introduce experiential learning activities right from the onset. The use of role playing or 'reality practice' was adapted as a technique for training in the various behavioural skills, especially those involving interpersonal relationships. This technique proved very useful during the six

165

Figure 7.7: Introduction to psychiatric nursing skills (Introductory Course — Pilot Study)

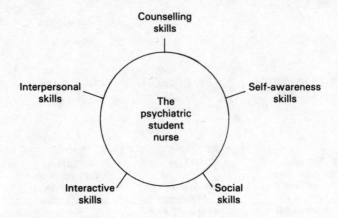

weeks of the Introductory Course, because it provided the opportunity to observe, practise and critically review the results of practice through discussion. It therefore allowed the learners to acquire skills in interaction with others by interacting, rather than by reading about it or by means of a lecture.

One such experience was aimed to developing intrapersonal and interpersonal skills, and, significant for the pilot-study, was developed and introduced during week 1 of the Introductory Course. This exercise involved the six learners undertaking a project on 'interviewing skills' (information-gathering skills — Figure 7.5). Each learner was asked to interview two 'key' members within the hospital's organisational structure (i.e. consultant, senior nurse, adminstrator, etc.) in order to identify their roles within it. This was a change from the previous format, where 'key' members from the hospital were invited to talk on their roles to groups in the Introductory Course as part of their orientation programme. It was felt that such an exercise would provide the opportunity to discuss the interviewing process in practice interviews and to evaluate the success and failure of individuals, and those of others in the group, in an environment in which the individuals would feel secure.

Prior to introducing this exercise the learners were provided with a general introduction to nursing models, followed by an overview of Peplau's (1952) interpersonal model of nursing. The learners were encouraged to participate in the learning process to explore the key issues pertaining to Peplau's model, for example:

166

(1) Peplau's concept of nursing;
(2) the role of the psychiatric nurse; and
(3) her four interpersonal phases and their relationship, leading to a logical progression of the nurse–patient relationship and the nursing process in psychiatric nursing.

This helped to lay the foundation for the development of inter-personal and intrapersonal skills, and to provide the opportunity to facilitate an experiential learning workshop on awareness of inter-personal skills. This workshop would provide the opportunity to reinforce some of the 'key' issues identified in Peplau's model, and would help in promoting peer support and group identity.

The next stage in preparing the learners for this exercise was the application of role playing to interviewer training. One learner was asked to play the part of a respondent, identifying herself with some actual person whom she knew, and to respond to the interviewer in terms of the role that she was playing. Another learner from the group was asked to play the role of interviewer. The remaining four learners were asked to act as observers. When the role-playing session ended, there was a general discussion of the techniques which the interviewer had used, the problems posed by the respon-dent, and the strengths and weaknesses which were demonstrated in fostering interpersonal skills development.

Such an exercise, facilitated through role playing, allows the learner who is playing the interviewer role to get the benefit of prac-ticising directly the words and techniques she must use in the inter-view situation. She will also get the experience of facing real problems without real consequences; that is, the exercise has reality, but she is not playing 'for keeps'. As a result, she is freer in her approach, and more able to observe herself than she would be in an actual interview situation.

The respondent also gets much out of playing her role, because she can perceive where the interviewer had failed to get information that was potentially available, and when the interviewer used tech-niques that were irritating. This may also provide self-awareness in the respondent, because she can analyse her own reactions to being interviewed and experience directly the effects of different inter-viewing techniques. Those who participate as observers will also have a chance to see the role playing in a more detached way and to plan the elimination of errors in their own interview techniques.

Following this preparation, the learners were given instruction to plan, negotiate and carry out the project assigned to them. They were allocated 2 hours each week to organise their project work, and 6 hours were allocated in week 6 for the learners to present their work to their peers and course tutors. The only tool given to the learners was a set of guidelines on interviewing skills technique to be referred to when planning the interviews, but arrangements for making appointments to carry out the interviews were left to the learners. The rationale for assigning this project to the Introductory Course learners was:

(1) to allow the learners to become familiar with the roles of 'key' hospital workers and the environment;
(2) to allow the learners to exercise autonomy;
(3) to engender an awareness of Peplau's interpersonal model of nursing; and
(4) to lay the foundation for the development of communication skills, particularly in the area of intrapersonal and interpersonal skills.

During the six weeks of the Introductory Course, a total of 65 hours was devoted to experiential learning exercises for the facilitation of psychiatric nursing skills development. The rest of the time was devoted to the broad areas selected from the knowledge base.

At the end of the Introductory Course, the learners were allocated for a period of 10 weeks to wards that offered experience in acute psychiatric care. Two learners were allocated to the psychiatric unit and the remaining four to the wards in the main hospital. During this allocation, tutorial support and guidance were provided in the form of ward-based tutorials/discussions and demonstrations once a week. At the end of 10 weeks the learners returned to the school of nursing to consolidate their experience and to complete this module.

Pilot study — discussion of findings (interpersonal skills development)

The discussion here is based on findings from formative and summative evaluations carried out during the pilot study.

(a) 'Off-job' (teaching content and teaching method)

A non-directive method was used to evaluate the overall teaching content of the Introductory Course. The learners were each asked to write on a blank sheet of paper their reaction to the teaching content.

All the six learners stated that, on the whole, the course achieved its stated aims and objectives, and covered the broad areas of the syllabus. They felt that the variety of teaching methods used during the 6 weeks facilitated the integration of the knowledge base from the different disciplines, and made it more meaningful, contextual and relative. They found Peplau's interpersonal model of nursing very interesting, and requested further input of her model in future modules. Four learners commented that an awareness of Peplau's model helped them considerably during their exercise in interviewing skills. They felt that it helped them identify their own strengths and weaknesses and those of their interviewees during the process of interaction. Some valuable comments were made regarding the sequencing and timing allocated for some of the teaching content.

Although there was general consensus on the use of a variety of teaching methods, one learner expressed reservations on experiential exercises and questioned the value of the exercise on interviewing skills. However, there was general approval of the use of the learners' past experiences during problem-solving activities which apparently enhanced their self-awareness skills.

There was praise for the tutors, and the learners enjoyed being seen as mature adults by the teaching staff. Three learners who had worked as nursing assistants before commencing nurse training felt that the andragogical approach by the teaching staff could be a maturing force in the learning process.

Evaluation of project work — 'interviewing skills'. The evaluation of interpersonal skills is a problem because it deals with human behaviour and interrelationships, which create variables that are difficult to control. Written assessments are not appropriate here, and reliable tools for measuring the response in an interaction situation are necessary. Therefore, in an attempt to experiment with self- and peer evaluation, two sets of questionnaires were devised, with four areas of concern. The questions related to:

(1) interviewing skills;
(2) teacher/student interpersonal relationships;
(3) attitude towards exercises on interviewing skills; and
(4) the peer-group relationships.

This type of formative evaluation allowed learners to write about and discuss their behaviour during the time the exercise was undertaken, thus identifying their strengths and weaknesses. The learners preferred this type of evaluation for identifying interpersonal skills

169

development; however, more work is needed before these methods can be 'institutionalised' into the curriculum. Furthermore, there was an overwhelming attraction towards experientially orientated activities, and the learners apparently enjoyed their interviewing exercise. They thought that it was a good way to gain confidence and assertiveness. They all appeared to have valued the opportunity to test some of the key concepts of Peplau's model as an introduction to interpersonal skills development.

(b) 'On-job' (first ward experience)

In order to evaluate this experience, a questionnaire, 'Evaluation of Clinical Experience', from the Joint Board of Clinical Nursing Studies Evaluation Package was adapted and used during the consolidation module. The results were somewhat alarming, and disappointing to say the least, but not so unexpected in the light of the anomaly that exists between theory and practice within the training institution. The following is a summary of the findings of this evaluation.

(1) Five out of six learners did not receive any formal orientation to the ward.

(2) Only two learners had opportunities to discuss their learning objectives.

(3) All six learners indicated that there was no correlation of theory and practice. Opportunities to try out some of their 'off-job' activities were not made available, even following attempts to request these. The learners, generally, experienced resistance from ward managers, and were constantly reminded that they were there to do some work. Two learners who confronted their ward managers were told, 'You are here to do a day's work, and there is no time for playing games! The school is the place to play games, and half the time the teachers don't know what goes on here. They should come here and see the real world, with real patients instead of preaching high-powered stuff!' All six learners expressed disappointment with their experience, and one learner stated that she was considering leaving nursing.

(4) Only one learner had any formal teaching, which was a lecture on electro-convulsive treatment. The only discussions/ demonstrations that were of any value were those facilitated by nurse teachers during their weekly sessions and those carried out by senior student nurses.

(5) The learners were critical of the 'handover' from one shift to

another. This lasted for only about 20 minutes on average, and was rooted very much in the 'medical model', with emphasis being placed on signs and symptoms, medical diagnosis, and medical treatments.

(6) None of the learners participated in case conferences, medical reviews, or multi-disciplinary meetings.

(7) None of the learners was assigned to care for an individual patient, or a group of patients. Instead, they were assigned to tasks for all the patients.

(8) None of the learners was regularly supported or supervised by mentors/preceptors due to low staffing levels and a singular lack of qualified staff.

(9) All six learners commented that 'new skills' were never demonstrated to them, practised under supervision or checked for competence. Comments also indicate that they were just told to get on with it!

(10) The final point is best demonstrated with the words of three of these learners on their overall reaction to their first ward experience:

'I feel the training ward could be better organised in its care for patients and teaching of student nurses, to ensure objectives are achieved.'

'I feel qualified staff should have some refresher courses, and the attitude of some staff leaves much to be desired. It is them who need training in interpersonal skills, not us!'

'I consider the ward [where] I did my acute admission experience unsuitable for a training ward, with little interest being shown by qualified staff and a very secretive atmosphere!'

The purpose of the Pilot Study was to examine the teaching content (1982 Mental Nursing Syllabus) and teaching method of interpersonal skills, and to determine the value of the learners' first practical experience for the enhancement and development of these skills. The results of the 'off-job' activities appeared favourable, and met the overall aims and objectives. However, the learners' experience in practice turned out to be unfavourable and disappointing.

The preparation of learners in specific psychiatric nursing skills did not match their practical experience. This was largely due to the lack of learning opportunities and support from qualified nurse preceptors/mentors. There appeared to be a significant shortfall in the integration of theory and practice, which caused considerable frustration and unsolicited anxiety in the learners.

171

DISCUSSION

The Pilot Study provided the tool to review the process of curriculum change in the light of our evaluation. The learners' contribution in evaluating the Introductory Course enabled us to review its theoretical framework, resulting in the preparation of a completely revised package for future Introductory Courses.

The learners' comments regarding the learning environment (wards) did give cause for concern, and immediate action was taken to renegotiate strategies for change within the learning environment. The anomaly between theory and practice is perhaps the single most critical problem facing psychiatric nursing, which Clinton (1981) states would be a singular factor in the failure of the 1982 Syllabus, but this should not impede curricular activities. Stenhouse (1975), for instance, refers to curriculum study as concerned with the relationship between the two views of curriculum — as *intention* and as *reality*. Educational realities seldom conform to our educational intentions, but this should not be viewed as failure, nor be regarded as peculiar to schools and teachers. Gott (1984) postulated that the different value systems between teacher and nurse practitioners make teachers work with an ideal model of care. This is certainly true in our case, where the value system among practitioners in the clinical areas is firmly rooted in a medical model of care, and is traditional and custodial in approach. The educational needs of learners are secondary to their service requirement. Gott found that the apprenticeship system of training was not even in evidence since learners often worked with other learners or untrained staff. This was a significant feature in our own evaluation of the Pilot Study.

In response to this anomaly, we decided to increase and improve ward-based teaching, something Reynolds and Cormack advocate in Chapter 6. Teachers allocated to specific areas of the clinical environment were encouraged to act as 'role models' for practitioners to develop psychiatric nursing skills. A reassessment of continuing education programmes was initiated, and further experientially orientated workshops were facilitated for nurse practitioners. Several 'on-the-job' training schemes were programmed, and are still in progress, for the facilitation of interpersonal, counselling, teaching and supervisory skills. The wards chosen to provide practical experience were further rationalised, so that fewer wards with adequate staffing levels are used for the implementation of the 1982 Syllabus. This was negotiated and decided jointly with senior service managers. The situation in the clinical environment, since the days of the Pilot Study, is favourable and has improved considerably, but needs monitoring and periodic evaluation.

The choice of using experiential learning exercises for inter-personal and self-awareness skills is in response to its prescription in the 1982 Syllabus, which bears a lot of resemblance to Peplau's model of nursing, and we feel that her model is just right for our curricular activities. It fits the changing role of the psychiatric nurse, and fosters the development of interpersonal relationships, a key role of the psychiatric nurse. Peplau's model could also be of value to other types of nursing where nurse–patient interaction is possible, but will not be suitable when dealing with an unconscious patient or an infant or in situations where the patient cannot respond to care. Her model also cannot be used in situations where the patient is a consumer of health education programmes through the use of mass media, where communication is one way! Since her theory deals with human behaviour and interrelationships, it is difficult to control variables. This requires reliable tools for measuring responses in an interaction situation, and therefore could pose problems when evaluating interpersonal skills. Peplau's model also lends itself to integration with a more recent model developed by King (1971), who perceives nursing as a dynamic process of actions, reactions, interactions and transactions, involving knowledge of the individual, social systems, perceptions, interpersonal relationships and health.

The curricular activities within the school of nursing are still in the Time-2 stage (Bolam, 1975); curriculum planning and develop-ment of the 1982 Syllabus are now advanced, and the completed document has now been submitted to the validating body (the English National Board).

The process of change is not without its problems. The success of innovation depends on maximising resources, material and personnel up to their fullest potential. Planning curricular activities has to be rational, and involve setting a timetable of events and monitoring progress of the objectives set. However, the most important factor influencing successful curriculum planning and development are effective communication with those involved in the process of change, an educationally supportive environment, and a sound knowledge of the subject.

REFERENCES

Bennis, W., Berne, K. and Chinn, R. (1970) *The planning of change*. Holt, Rinehart & Winston, London.

Bloom, B.S. (ed.) (1979) *Taxonomy of educational objectives: the classification of educational goals. Handbook I: Cognitive domain*. McKay, New York.

Bobbit, F. (1981) *The curriculum*. Houghton Mifflin, Boston

Bolam, R. (1975) The management of educational change: towards a conceptual framework, in R. Houghton *et al.* (eds) *Management in Education*. Open University, Ward Lock Educational, London

Chater, S.S. (1975) A conceptual framework for curriculum development. *Nursing Outlook, 23* (7), 428–33.

Clinton, M.E. (1981) Training psychiatric nurses: a sociological study of the problem of integrating theory and practice, unpublished PhD thesis, University of East Anglia.

Derdiarian, A.K. (1979) Education: a way to theory construction in nursing. *Journal of Nursing Education, 18* (2), 36–47

English National Board (1982) *Syllabus of Training, Professional Register — Part 3. (Registered Mental Nurse)*. ENB, London

General Nursing Council (1974) Training syllabus: Register of Nurses, Mental Nursing. GNC for England and Wales, London

General Nursing Council (1982) Response to 'Draft' — 1981 Mental Nursing. (Circular 82/13) Syllabus of Training. GNC for England and Wales, London

General Nursing Council (1983) Educational policy document (Circular 83/13, June, 1983). GNC for England and Wales, London

Gott, M. (1984) *Learning Nursing*. Royal College of Nursing, Research Series. RCN, London

Harrow, A. (1972) *A taxonomy of psychomotor domain*. McKay, New York

King, I. (1971) *Towards a theory of nursing*. John Wiley, New York

Krathwohl, D.R., Bloom, B.S. and Masia, B.B. (1964) *Taxonomy of educational objectives: the classification of educational goals — Handbook II: affective domain*. McKay, New York

Nisbet, J. (1974) Innovation — bandwagon or hearse, in Harris *et al.* (eds) *Curriculum innovation*. Open University-Press, Milton Keynes

Nursing Theories Conference Group (1980) *Nursing Theories*. Prentice Hall, Englewood Cliffs, NJ

Peplau, H.E. (1952) *Interpersonal relations in nursing: a conceptual frame of reference for psychodynamic nursing*. Putnam, New York

Peplau, H.E. (1960) Talking with patients. *American Journal of Nursing, 60*, 964–6

Peplau, H.E. (1969) Professional closeness. *Nursing Forum, 8*, 343–59

Sparks, S.M., Vitalo, P.B., Cohen, B.F. and Kahn, G.S. Teaching of interpersonal skills to nurse practitioner students. *Journal of Continuing Education in Nursing, 11* (3), 5–15

Stenhouse, L. (1975) *An introduction to curriculum research and development*. Heinemann, London

Stevens, B.J. (1979) *Nursing theory*. Little, Brown, Boston

Tyler, K.W. (1949) *Basic principles of curriculum and instruction*. University of Chicago Press, Chicago, Ill.

Walton, M. (1983) *Management and managing: a dynamic approach*. Harper & Row, London

Wheeler, D.K. (1967) *Curriculum process*. Hodder & Stoughton, London

8

Teaching Psychology to Nurses

L.A. Wattley and D.J. Müller

This chapter describes a practical approach to teaching psychology to nurses in which students and teachers participate in psychological investigative procedures such as observation, interviewing and experimenting. All of these procedures are set in the context of nursing, and the topics that are selected for investigation introduce students to relevant research from both psychology and nursing. The general aim is for the students to learn psychological knowledge to help them with their work, and to understand how human behaviour is researched, thus encouraging the development of research-mindedness. Our method of teaching is set out in more detail in Wattley and Müller (1984). Here we will concentrate on some of the broader educational issues underlying this approach.

NEEDS AND PROBLEMS

The need for nurses to have knowledge from the behavioural sciences has been identified within nursing by researchers such as Birch (1979), who linked a lack of such knowledge with high levels of learner anxiety, and Gott (1984), who felt that learners were very inadequately prepared for the psychological as well as the practical skills demanded of a nurse. Historically, the inclusion of psychology into nurse education seems to have been only a vague requirement and rarely linked with nursing practice (Wattley and Müller, 1983a). It is obvious, however, from reading current syllabuses (e.g. General Nursing Council, 1977; University of London Diploma in Nursing, 1980, 1981), that the profession is committed to its inclusion at pre- and post-registration levels, and that increasingly it is thought that psychology should be concerned with nursing practice

176

(Crow, 1976; Clarke, 1981; King, 1984). However, various problems are experienced in trying to teach psychology at all. For example, many nurse educators feel insufficiently familiar with psychology to teach it (Birch, 1979), yet according to Wells (1983) few schools of nursing are able to employ psychologists to help. Similarly, few psychologists, at least initially, are very familiar with nursing. This leads to problems such as those described in a report by the British Psychological Society (1974) of teaching 'watered-down academic psychology' when nurses really want help with dealing with very stressful human situations (e.g. coping with pain, death, anxiety, etc.). Another problem can occur if clinical psychologists teach nurses but concentrate on abnormal psychology rather than 'health psychology', which may be more applicable to a wider range of nurses (Niven, 1982). These problems may perhaps be less acute in areas where links have been established between schools of nursing and institutions of higher or further education if these allow for some mutual sharing and exploring of needs and resources between nurses and psychologists. We suspect though that for many nurse educators a problem remains: whether or not they have access to helpful psychologists, the students have to be taught psychology, and since the syllabuses can be vague and curricula restricting, there are questions to be asked about *what* to teach, *how* to teach, *when* it should be taught, and by *whom*.

In this chapter we have addressed these problems by describing our own work in this field in some detail. Our ideas are drawn from our experience of teaching psychology to nurses at all levels including pre- and post-registration and graduate and postgraduate students. This work arose from our desire to meet two very important needs in nurse education which are reflected in the literature, and which we consider to be fundamentally linked. These are first to help nurses understand themselves and others better, which it is thought will enhance patient care and reduce nursing stress (Birch, 1975; Clarke, 1981; Gott, 1984); and secondly to encourage research-mindedness (Wattley and Müller, 1983a, b). This second need is increasingly viewed as an important aim, so that nursing can be a truly research-based profession. A scientific basis clearly enhances the professional status of nursing, and should contribute towards improved patient care. However, serious considerations should be given to the forceful argument put forward by Miller (1985) concerning the gap between theory and practice and the need to address this explicitly.

Psychology, a discipline similar in age to modern nursing, has retained during the past hundred years its commitment to research. Nursing, strangely and despite promising beginnings, did not. The need to forge stronger links between psychology and nursing has recently been reiterated in the American literature in an issue of the *American Psychologist* (DeLeon, Kjervik, Kraut and Van den Bos, 1985). Both disciplines are concerned with individuals, and therefore their focus is the same and the methods of studying humans which have been developed in the behavioural sciences and especially in psychology are of immense value to nurses.

This usefulness is important in at least two ways. First, learning *what* psychologists have discovered about human behaviour can help nurses understand various aspects of their work much better. However, experience and research (BPS, 1974) has suggested to us that learning content alone is not always effective. We consider it to be more helpful, interesting and less mysterious to teach nurses at the same time how the knowledge from psychology was arrived at. This enables us to teach nurses the complexities and controversies underlying this knowledge, even though this creates uncertainty (Shepherd, Durham and Foot, 1976). The alternative tends to be to present nurses with broad generalisations which may be misleading or inaccurate. This approach fails to show that research serves to throw further light on to previous ideas and helps change our understanding of human behaviour accordingly. Thus, in the long run, presenting nurses with 'facts' alone is more confusing than developing their awareness over time of the existence of uncertainty in all areas of knowledge, and the contribution of research towards our enlightenment. Introducing uncertainty also allows for discussion of how to act in spite of it.

Secondly, learning *how* psychologists have investigated human behaviour introduces nurses to learning research techniques relevant to their work. As a result, they are able to develop skills in critical thinking, to understand the need for measurement, to use the research literature and to learn ways of carrying out objective investigations. This may sound unrealistic for the majority of nurses, yet the process of nursing is also scientific in its intent, expecting nurses to identify problems, plan how they can be resolved, and evaluate the success of their plans. It is doubtful whether nurses are adequately prepared for these skills, especially where they involve collecting information about patient behaviour, for example attitudes or reactions to illness which are essentially psychological components of the totality of nursing care. Our primary purpose then in designing this method of teaching psychology was to teach *process* as well as content, in other words, ways in which psychological knowledge is gained as well as the psychology knowledge *per se*.

SPECIFIC CONSIDERATIONS

Various considerations guide our selection of material to be included in what we teach using this approach. First, the subject matter should be relevant to nursing. This view is self-evident and strongly supported in the literature (cf. BPS, 1974; Pratt, 1979; King, 1984). The temptation to limit psychology to its pure and theoretical under-pinnings is strongly criticised in the context of nursing, at least in courses for non-specialists. As has been discussed elsewhere (Müller, Harris and Wattley, 1986), applied psychology must, to some extent, be prescriptive and encourage the trying out of ideas and knowledge in practice. In our own work we have used this criterion of relevance as a major determinant of content. Thus, for example, we have included practicals on nurses' personality and their recruitment to the profession; on the significance of life events such as becoming a parent; on interpersonal perception including stereotyping of patients; on the role of memory in co-operating with treatment; and on the nurses' work situation. This list serves to illustrate a range of content, but it is not exhaustive.

This limitation on content brings us to a second vitally important consideration, which is that the method of teaching must be compat-ible with ethical principles. Since our method involves the students in carrying out practicals, it is important to ensure that they can do so without contravening the ethics of nursing, psychology or research. Thus they use each other or friends as subjects, but not colleagues while at work, nor, of course, patients. Such investiga-tions require the consent of ethical committees, thus extending the scope of this teaching method beyond its original intention and being not in keeping with the nature of the exercises. This limited exposure to the principles of ethical behaviour in research and in nursing is important not just in terms of understanding psychology, but also in serving to prepare nurses to make sound judgements about the nature of research requests which they may encounter at work, and to protect patients and staff. Thus, although the explicit aim may be to teach psychological methods and knowledge, there are implicit opportunities for enhancing nursing education more generally.

A third consideration is to provide a range of techniques from the behavioural sciences which give nurses insight into the methods of data collection in psychology. In our book (Wattley and Müller, 1984) we have presented 17 practicals ranging from highly prepared and structured exercises, to those demanding much more creativity on the part of the student. We have included five main types of research methods representing those that are particularly appropriate to the psychology topics included in each chapter: observation; interviews, questionnaires and rating scales; experiments; descriptive techniques such as content analysis; and experiential techiques such as role play. In carrying these out, nurses can begin to discover what sort of difficulties are encountered in investigating human behaviour. The apparatus required consists only of pen, paper and a watch with a second hand. Simple analysis and discussion of results takes place in the light of the chapter introductions which describe recent research appropriate to the topic. Students are encouraged to follow up references for themselves and to write up the practicals to get the feel for the way research is reported and to help them find their way around published material. Results are not tested statistically for significance, though able students and undergraduates could move on to this more demanding aspect if need be.

PRACTICAL EXAMPLES

The best way of describing our method of teaching psychology to nurses is to give examples of some of the practicals we have used. We have selected three practicals illustrative of the range of topics and techniques covered.

Teaching psychological methods of research serves to introduce nurses to both quantitative and qualitative methods, which are both appropriate for nurses to appreciate since nursing is described by Orr (1979) as being at the interface between physical and social sciences. Psychology does embrace both the 'harder' and the 'softer' elements of research approaches, and this can be useful in helping nurses to become research-minded in the widest sense applicable to their work.

Communication

The topic of communication is important in nursing, and efforts are being made in many areas to provide social or interpersonal skills training to nurses (cf. Kagan, 1985; Kagan, Evans and Kay, 1986). Other factors affecting communication can be studied, however, such as memory. Much concern is expressed over the failure of patients to co-operate with medical advice, and this has been investigated in detail. One paper, for example, by Ley (1979), reviews a range of particularly relevant research concerned with improving memory for advice. However, nurses are also expected to remember a lot of information. In one of our practicals, nurses compare themselves with regard to their ability to recall or recognise the names of drugs. This has implications for themselves ('Never take a telephone prescription, nurse') and for their patients, especially somebody being discharged who may need to remember a variety of drug names and instructions. In the practical, a class of students is divided into two groups and given a list of ten drug names to memorise during a 45-second period. Then half the group are asked to write down what they remember, and half are presented with a random list of drugs including all those which they were asked to memorise and quite a few more. All this group has to do is underline the original ten. The practical takes only a few minutes but the results are usually quite dramatic and clearly indicate how error creeps in for the 'recall' group as well as failure to remember all the items. The 'recognition' group on the other hand rarely make a mistake and tend to remember all ten names.

Such a practical serves several purposes. It introduces students to relevant and recent research; it demonstrates important implications for their clinical practice (and discussion can be encouraged to explore this further); it presents an opportunity to compare their own performance with those of other groups doing the same practical (we give data of our own for comparison in each practical); and it encourages critical discussion and the creation of new ways of testing hypotheses, such as the notion that senior nurses do better because drug names are more familiar. A further useful discovery for nurses can be the relevance of psychology to themelves and their own behaviour, not just their patients. Depending on time or other factors, this practical can be used simply as an illustration for a lecture on psychology, communication, or nursing practice; or as one of several practicals designed to explore the role that memory might play in communication. There is, therefore, plenty of scope for explaining 'content' alongside the 'process' of the practical. Since the 'process' is experimental, students can begin to explore the problems as well as the advantages of this kind of method for understanding human behaviour in the nursing context.

Nursing image

The public image of nursing is topical and of concern to many nurses, as revealed by Murray (1983) who linked it with some nurses' intention to leave nursing. In our practical, which is based on Murray's original work, the students rate themselves according to a number of characteristics such as how shy they are or how sympathetic. They do this on a five-point scale between two extremes, e.g. shy → confident, sympathetic → unsympathetic. Some time later they complete an identical scale, this time considering what the public expects them to be like. A further set of data can be collected by the students asking members of the public to complete the same scale (again an opportunity to discuss ethical considerations).

When we have run this practical we have found our results to be comparable with Murray's: nurses believe that the public expect a great deal of them, and, although their own self-image is quite high, it does not match these expectations. We also found that what the public actually think of nurses is much more similar to the nurses' own view of themselves than to their imagined public expectations.

This practical serves to introduce nurses to psychology which is directly relevant to them and their career. We chose also to include 'content' about absence and wastage problems linked to studies of stress in nursing. These illustrate to nurses the fact that relevant research is going on and may increase their awareness of the causes of problems among carers at work. Similarly, it introduces the use of a rating scale as a means of eliciting information. Its value, or problems experienced in completing it, can be discussed, and this hopefully will help nurses to be aware of the implications of this kind of method when they read research based on such techniques.

Stress in patients

One of the key issues in nursing at the present time seems to be stress, both in nurses and in patients. It is a difficult concept to define and measure, but it has been suggested that its presence can affect outcome in the clinical setting. For example, stress expressed as anxiety was found by Boore (1978) to affect recovery rate in surgical patients. Johnston (1982) has found that nurses tend to overestimate what patients worry about, and though they know in general terms the kinds of things that concern patients, they are not good at identifying the specific worries of individual patients. One of our practicals introduces nurses to some research by Volicer and Bohannon (1975) which gives patients' rank orders of events that they consider stressful in hospital. The practical is devised to enable nurses to try to predict how patients would rank-order these events, and to compare their individual and group scores with those of the patients in the original study. In this way they can see which stressors they tend to overestimate, which they underestimate, and which they rate equally with the patients. They can also compare themselves with other groups of nurses, e.g. intensive care nurses, qualified nurses, student nurses, and even non-nurses if they are prepared to collect such data and can do so in an appropriate and ethical manner. We tend to keep data from different classes and pass on the information for comparison.

The practical is a useful way of helping nurses to explore the concept of stress in practice as viewed by patients and themselves. The method is similar to that of Holmes and Rahe (1967) and is therefore useful for explaining the way that 'life-event scores' are obtained. The practical can serve as an introduction to more factual psychological research into stress, or to further study of relevant nursing research. Depending on the level and needs of the students it can be used simply as an indicator of differences between patients' and nurses' perceptions of the same events, or as a means of understanding in much more depth how stress research might be done.

CONSUMERS OF PSYCHOLOGY

'Talk and chalk' methods of teaching psychology to nurses have been quite rightly criticised (BPS, 1974). The practicals we have described are intended to help students develop an active under-standing of the relevance of psychology to their work. We would argue that our method is an appropriate introduction to psychology in the context of nursing, in that it introduces nurses to relevant resource material from both psychological and nursing research. This means that nurses can quickly become familiar with this sort of material, and can begin to take their own interests and needs further. Hopefully, this encourages them to want to find things out for themselves and gives them confidence in handling the various sources. This may mean too that they can cope better where more traditional teaching methods are employed and make more use of such material according to their own needs.

In taking this approach we are acknowledging too that it may not be incumbent upon teachers to teach nurses everything from psychology which it is felt they need to know. In an ideal situation it would make educational sense to use our methods of teaching as an introduction in pre-registration courses, to be followed up by more specific study according to the level of nursing experience at the time later on in initial training. Having learned some principles concerned with how behaviour is investigated and where information can be obtained, students should find it easier to make further use of psychological knowledge in relation to their work. Demystifying the ways in which psychological knowledge is obtained makes it more accessible to the people who look to the discipline for help with the problems encountered in their daily work. In proposing this approach to teaching psychology, our intention is to help nurses to become consumers of psychology, in such a way that they can consult appropriate resources and draw from them the help they seek for their work. The resources may be literature and research, or psychologists themselves. Llewellyn and Fielding (1983), for example, have written a twelve-part series in the *Nursing Mirror* spelling out the practical ways in which psychologists can help nurses actually in clinical areas such as mental handicap, intensive therapy units, psychiatry and so on.

Our second stated aim is the development of research-mindedness, and we have described why we feel our teaching methods can help attain this goal. It is worth pointing out that although research-mindedness is to be encouraged, it does not necessarily imply that these individuals are capable of carrying out or even implementing research. In the first case, much more training and more sophisticated approaches will be required before a person can contemplate carrying out research, and this is rarely an activity for an individual alone. All researchers need to work closely with others. In the second case, implementing findings must always be a group or team concern, drawing on nursing and psychological expertise involving other staff. It requires a great deal of literature searching, discussion and ongoing evaluation, and again is not an activity for an individual nurse working alone. Lelean (1980) following up the Briggs Report (1972) argues that there are at least three levels of nurse in the context of research; the researcher who is highly trained, the assistant who may be helping an experienced researcher, and the remainder, who should be research-minded. Research-mindedness is an attitude of mind expressed in one's approach to knowledge.

TEACHING PSYCHOLOGY PRACTICALS

So far we have explored what aspects of psychology to teach and the teaching methods that might be adopted. We have not prescribed the content of a course, but have offered a structure to serve at an introductory level with implications for subsequent learning related to the future needs of nurses. We now turn briefly to the questions of when to teach psychology and who might do it.

When to teach psychology practicals

There are two sides to this question: when in a nurse's education should practicals be introduced; and at what point in a particular course. We have found from our experience that nurses can be introduced to psychology early on in their initial training by using our approach. In practice we find ourselves teaching this way at all pre- and post-registration levels, and as long as one is aware of any psychology already understood or familiar to the students, it is easy to draw on their current knowledge in relation to the practicals. One may choose to emphasise a particular methodology rather than the psychological topic if appropriate. Nurses have rarely if ever in our experience described this approach as unwelcome or repetitive of earlier knowledge.

Similarly, when to teach psychology practicals may be affected by the particular aims of the course in progress. For example, we used this method in the first year of the University of Wales Diploma in Nursing as preparation for a research project required of the students in the third year. On another course, undergraduate first-year students studying for a Bachelor of Nursing degree were introduced to psychology by means of a lecture on alternate weeks with illustrative practicals in between. In some cases we have given 'one-off' practicals, say to a group of nurses doing an intensive care course, in order to demonstrate some aspect of psychology, why it may be relevant, and how it can be measured. The key is probably to be flexible. If timetabling-in a whole course is inappropriate for some reason, the method need not be rejected as it lends itself to 'one-off' situations.

Psychological practicals then can be taught at times to suit the particular course in question. If it is possible to make them available as an introduction to psychology, there may be advantages especially in helping students seek specific psychological knowledge for

185

themselves early on in their education. Developing research-mindedness may also help make them more discerning consumers of the knowledge available and help them acquire a more enquiring approach towards the knowledge base necessary for nursing. Learning psychology is something which ideally should continue throughout a nurse (or teacher's) career.

Who should teach psychology practicals

Our book was designed so that students could if necessary be their own teachers. Psychologists without nursing knowledge may find it useful for developing their own awareness of the application of psychology to nursing, and, having established some ground work with students from the practicals, may find it easier to go on to more familiar territory. Nurse teachers on the other hand may find the book helpful for enhancing their own knowledge of some psychology so that students can then take more initiative themselves according to their interests. Our approach is not intended to be seen as all that nurses need to know in psychology, but it does try to offer some solutions to the real problems of knowing what to teach, when and by whom, bearing in mind the situation described at the beginning of the chapter. Teachers may also be interested in a resource book for teachers of psychology, Rose and Radford (1984), which details other materials such as audiovisual packages that are available to help. Psychology may be taught by different people within the same course, and therefore we think that providing nurses with some preparation to enable them to become consumers of psychology, if necessary without skilled teaching, is worth while. We hope that our method achieves this.

OVERVIEW

There is a final more controversial point which needs raising. The rationale for teaching nurses psychology hinges on the premise that in the long run it will improve patient care. What is being argued, then, is that through the inclusion of psychology in the nursing curriculum, nurses will become better equipped for their jobs. One of the problems in supporting this viewpoint is that it is difficult to evaluate in a concrete way the contribution that psychology makes. Certainly, it is relatively easy to assess the learners' progress through the more traditional means of assessment, such as essays, projects and examinations. Yet in doing this we must ask whether this measures in any way the nurses' ability to integrate psychology into their daily work.

In the long term it might be possible to evaluate the contribution nurses with psychological training make to developing research. But in the short term it is our view that some attempt should be made to include psychology more in the clinical training of nurses. After studying and practising communication skills we would expect nurses to transfer their knowledge to the ward situation or wherever they are working. One would expect a knowledge of the psychological aspects of hospitalisation for children to influence how nurses interact with both parents and children while the latter are in hospital. An understanding of the psychological factors affecting recovery after surgery should result in more sensitive patient care. These significant effects from learning psychology need to be evaluated in the context in which they are expected to occur. There is clearly no better place than the nurse's own work environment. In order to achieve this successfully, psychologists need to develop even more sensitive measures of how psychology can be successfully applied in practice. On the other hand, the nursing profession itself might benefit from encouraging more involvement by psychologists in the work setting. Hopefully, these two developments will occur in conjunction with each other, and we can look forward to an even more fruitful collaboration between nursing and psychology in the future.

REFERENCES

Birch, J. (1975) *To nurse or not to nurse.* Royal College of Nursing, London

Birch, J. (1979) The anxious learners. *Nursing Mirror*, 13 February, 17–22

Boore, J. (1978) *Prescription for recovery.* Royal College of Nursing, London

Briggs, A. (1972) *Report of the Committee on Nursing.* HMSO, London

British Psychological Society (1974) Teaching psychology to nurses. *Bulletin of the British Psychological Society, 27*, 272–83

Clarke, M. (1981) Two aspects of psychology and their applications to nursing, in J.P. Smith (ed.) *Nursing science in nursing practice.* Butterworths, London

Crow, R.A. (1976) A fresh look at psychology in nursing. *Journal of Advanced Nursing, 1*, 51–62

DeLeon, P.H., Kjervik, D.K., Kraut, A.G. and Van den Bos, G.R. (1985)

Psychology and nursing: a natural alliance. *American Psychologist, 40* (11), 1153–64

General Nursing Council (1977) *Training syllabus: Register of General Nursing.* General Nursing Council, London

Gott, M. (1984) *Learning nursing.* Royal College of Nursing, London

Holmes, T.H. and Rahe, R.H. (1967) The social readjustment rating scale. *Journal of Psychosomatic Research, 11,* 213–18

Johnston, M. (1982) Recognition of patients' worries by nurses and by other patients. *British Journal of Clinical Psychology, 21,* 255–61

Kagan, C.M. (ed.) (1985) *Interpersonal skills in nursing. Research and applications.* London, Croom Helm

Kagan, C., Evans, J. and Kay, B. (1986) *A manual of interpersonal skills for nurses: an experiential approach.* Harper & Row, London

King, J. (1984) Striking it right: psychology in nursing, four-part series. *Nursing Times,* 17, 24, 31 October, 7 November

Lelean, S. (1980) Research in nursing: 1. *Nursing Times Occasional Papers, 76* (2), 5–8

Ley, P. (1979) Memory for medical information. *British Journal of Social and Clinical Psychology, 18,* 151–4

Llewellyn, S. and Fielding, G. (1983) Psychology series, parts 1–12, *Nursing Mirror,* 9 February–27 April

Miller, A. (1985) The relationship between nursing theory and nursing practice. *Journal of Advanced Nursing, 10,* 417–24

Müller, D.J., Harris, P. and Wattley, L.A. (1986) *Nursing children: psychology, research and practice.* Harper & Row, London

Murray, M. (1983) Role conflict and intention to leave nursing. *Journal of Advanced Nursing, 8,* 29–31

Niven, N. (1982) Health psychology. *Nursing Times,* 10 March, 417–19

Orr, J.A. (1979) Nursing and the process of scientific enquiry. *Journal of Advanced Nursing, 4,* 603–10

Pratt, J. (1979) Teaching psychology in health studies courses. *Journal of Further and Higher Education, 3,* 56–9

Rose, D. and Radford, J. (eds) (1984) *Teaching psychology. Information and resources.* British Psychological Society, Leicester

Shepherd, G., Durham, R. and Foot, D. (1976) Teaching psychology to nurses: suggestions for a new course. *Bulletin of the British Psychological Society, 29,* 45–8

University of London (1980) *Diploma in Nursing: proposals for a new course*

University of London (1981) Diploma in Nursing. Revised syllabus

Volicer, J. and Bohannon, M.W. (1975) A hospital stress rating scale. *Nursing Research, 24,* 352–9

Wattley, L.A. and Müller, D.J. (1983a) Psychology and nursing: the case for an empirical approach. *Journal of Advanced Nursing, 8,* 107–10

Wattley, L.A. and Müller, D.J. (1983b) Towards a psychology of nursing. *Journal of Advanced Nursing, 8,* 341–2

Wattley, L.A. and Müller, D.J. (1984) *Investigating psychology: a practical approach for nursing.* Harper & Row, London

Wells, J.C. (1983) Critique of 'Psychology and nursing: the case for an empirical approach'. *Journal of Advanced Nursing, 8,* 339–41

9

Communication Skills Teaching in Nurse Education

J. Macleod Clark and A. Faulkner

INTRODUCTION

There have been many descriptive research studies of communication patterns between nurses and patients, e.g. Faulkner (1980), Ashworth (1980) and Macleod Clark (1982). Such studies usefully identified deficiencies in nurses' ability to communicate effectively with their patients, and raised a number of issues regarding the reasons for nurses' deficits. However, descriptive studies do not produce answers to problems; rather they point the way to future research. This chapter deals with more recent research into the area of communication in nursing which arose primarily from the findings of researchers such as Faulkner and Macleod Clark who both suggested that more emphasis should be put on teaching communication skills in the basic nurse training curriculum.

Three questions immediately arise. The first is concerned with tutors and their attitudes towards and knowledge of communication skills; the second is concerned with the priority given to teaching these skills; and the third concerns the effect that teaching communication skills can have on the learners themselves.

In 1980, the Health Education Council (HEC) funded the Communication in Nurse Education (CINE) project. The prime purpose was to develop an effective means of helping nurses to develop the basic communication skills which are an essential prerequisite to taking on an active health education role in nursing. The project was designed with the aim of teaching basic communication skills to nurse learners in the first 18 months of basic general training, and then evaluating the programme by using a pre-test, post-test design (Campbell and Stanley, 1966) and control groups.

In addition to this, the question of communication in the

curriculum was addressed by means of two national surveys, one of Directors of Nurse Education (DNEs) and one of nurse tutors. The DNE survey would precede the teaching programme for student nurses and would be used to identify schools of nursing willing to take part in the CINE project. Detailed information about the questionnaires and results of the surveys can be found in the project report (CINE, 1986).

THE DNE SURVEY

The aim of the survey was to identify in each school the commitment to teaching specific communication skills courses, the place of teaching communication skills within basic training and the attitudes held by DNEs towards communication. A questionnaire was designed and piloted on a small sample of DNEs who were asked to complete it and comment on its format and design. From this pilot it was found necessary to change one question and omit another.

All DNEs in England, Wales and Northern Ireland, except those taking part in the pilot study, were sent the revised questionnaire. There was an 84% response rate giving a representative view of how DNEs perceived communication as part of the curriculum.

THE TUTOR'S SURVEY

The questionnaire was modified for tutors where necessary. For example, where DNEs had been asked 'How well do you feel that tutors have been prepared to teach communication skills?', tutors were asked 'How well do you think *you* have been prepared to teach . . .' This modified questionnaire was sent to tutors in every school of nursing throughout Britain, addressed to the tutor responsible for teaching communications skills, with the invitation to complete a copy extended to other tutors involved in the subject. The 288 questionnaires returned represented 75% of schools of nursing in England, Wales and Northern Ireland, and all colleges of nursing in Scotland except two.

ANALYSIS OF QUESTIONNAIRES

In analysing the completed questionnaires it soon became obvious that there were high levels of agreement between DNEs and tutors about communication in the curriculum. The tutors' reponses, however, being at the grass roots, perhaps gave a more realistic picture of the problems related to putting the subject into the curriculum.

Commitment to teaching communication skills

Communication is taught both as a separate subject and within sessions on other subjects in most schools or colleges of nursing in Britain. However, most tutors are expected to teach across the full range of subjects in the curriculum, which could well raise issues of expertise in any one particular subject. In fact, 65% of Scottish tutors were actively engaged in teaching communication skills, with only 36% feeling they had had preparation for such teaching. In the rest of Britain 97% of tutors were actively engaged in the teaching but only 73% had had some training in teaching the subject. Overall, less than 5% of tutors felt that they were 'totally prepared' for such teaching. In this respect, DNEs were more pessimistic, suggesting that only 2% of staff were very well prepared for teaching communication skills.

Such findings raise a number of questions related to commitment to communication as part of the curriculum, not only for the teacher but also for the learners. James (1975) suggests that the effective teacher '. . . must be able to identify clearly the changes he wants to see in his learners'. He also suggests that '. . . for success in nurse education, teachers must be motivated to teach and learners to learn'. It is suggested here that if teachers are not 'experts' in teaching communication as a subject, they may well be unaware of what they should be formulating in terms of goals and objectives, and will almost certainly be unable to generate enthusiasm for the subject in their students.

In fact, both DNEs and tutors felt that it was very important for communication to be taught as a subject (87–95%), but, conversely, little time appears to be set aside for such teaching. Few DNEs and even fewer tutors thought that more than 10% of curriculum time was devoted to the subject, and many felt that less than 5% was a more realistic figure. This low priority may well equate to curricula which continue to be planned around medical specialities rather than to a patient-centred approach to teaching.

191

Teaching methods

A variety of methods are used for teaching communication skills, the major ones being role play and experiential teaching, the use of audiovisual material and discussion. Least used methods were written work, case studies, and ward-based teaching. This latter contrasts with a stated belief by a majority of both DNEs and tutors that the ward is the most appropriate place for communication to be taught. It may be that this belief is linked with the notion that ward staff should do such teaching. If this is the case, students may well fail to learn effective communication skills since Macleod Clark (1983) and Faulkner and Maguire (1984) found that trained nurses lack the basic skills required for professional communication.

The school or college of nursing was seen as the second most appropriate place for nurses to be taught communication in this respect, most being well equipped for such teaching in that over 90% have a full range of audio and audiovisual aids. There is, however, some indication that full use may not be made of these aids by all tutors. Most importantly, only half of the schools and colleges have the services of a technician. This means that there is no one to help tutors understand or use equipment, and that there is a lack of regular servicing and maintenance of the various aids.

Tutors were asked if there were limitations or constraints on the use of audiovisual equipment. Only 39% of tutors said that there were *no* limitations to its use, and it may be that many tutors may be loath to use it because of potential problems. Over 30% saw time as a major limitation, and this could well be linked to lack of a technician who could set up, test and dismantle equipment before and after a teaching session. There may also be a link with comments from 10% of the tutors who said that the equipment was poorly serviced, as equipment which is at risk of failing can erode valuable teaching time.

Some tutors (11%) felt that access to equipment was a problem, which may be linked with security problems, and others (10%) felt that their groups were too large for the audiovisual aids to be useful, this latter linking with problems of accommodation. Fifteen per cent of tutors felt that their own inexperience in using the equipment limited its use, and this again links with the lack of a technician and possibly with a lack of appropriate training in the use of audiovisual equipment. Overall, it appears that although schools and colleges are well equipped in regard to audiovisual aids, these are largely underused by the majority of staff. However, some tutors felt that there was not enough equipment. This was the major complaint of Scottish tutors, possibly related to the fact that only 70% had access to the full range of equipment as opposed to 95% in the rest of Britain.

Reading and resources

Commitment to a subject may also be judged by the reading material recommended to students, and the tutors' knowledge of available resources. Only 77% of the tutor sample in Scotland and 87% in the rest of Britain responded to the question, 'Which reading on communication do you recommend to your students'. Of those responding, many gave very vague answers. For example, 'current journals' gives no specific information, and books were often listed by title alone without any mention of author, publisher or year of publication.

Reading material listed fell into three broad categories, i.e. journals and journal articles, nursing texts, and non-nursing texts, of which psychology texts were in the majority. Some tutors listed specific journal articles such as 'The talking points series in *Nursing Times*', whereas others cited the journal alone, such as *Nursing Times* or *Nursing Mirror* or simply 'nursing journals'.

There were some differences between Scotland and the rest of Britain on the resouces used, and some ambivalence over what constituted a resource. One tutor simply stated, 'Meetings, bloody meetings' as a response, and another specified '*Nursing Times* journal'. Most other tutors referred to teaching aids such as the 'DHSS Caring Communication Package' or the 'Abbot' videos.

Courses

Given the above findings there is obviously a problem for tutors in relation to teaching communication skills. In view of the short time available for teaching, difficulty in using equipment, the tutors' lack of preparedness to teach and lack of knowledge on reading and resource materials, it can be suggested that some remedial action is necessary. Tutors were asked to suggest such action by stating which course they would like to attend to improve their communication skills teaching.

Many tutors felt that suitable courses did not exist at present but a few listed specific courses. As with reading and resource materials, there was a lack of detail from tutors with just a few exceptions. Table 9.1 shows specific courses listed by tutors. The need for courses can be seen to be particularly important since effective communication skills teaching involves the use of experiential teaching methods, audiovisual equipment and group work. In order to put these methods into practice it is essential that tutors have the knowledge, skill and confidence so that students can learn in an atmsophere of trust (Tomlinson, Macleod Clark and Faulkner, 1984). Indeed it is suggested that for an unprepared tutor to use such methods could be dangerous in emotional terms to both teacher and students, and that courses should be a mandatory prerequisite for communication skills teaching.

Table 9.1: A range of courses tutors would like to attend

Course	Organisers/venue	Tutors, Scotland	Tutors, England, Wales, Northern Ireland
Counselling skills for nurses	None given		*
Teaching methods and ideas	None given	*	*
Med. course — human relations	None given		
Workshops for teachers of nurses	ENB, RCN, London		
Teaching assertion	None given		
Interviewing skills	None given		
2-day course	Ripon College, York		
Microteaching skills	None given		
Social skills training	None given		
Transactional analysis	None given		
Advanced Makaton Bliss symbolics	None given		
King's Fund Counselling Course	GNC		
Short course, small study groups	Scottish Institute of Human Relations, Edinburgh		
Counselling	Scottish Association of Counselling		
Group dynamics	Richmond Fellowship course		

* = mentioned by more than one tutor

ATTITUDES TO COMMUNICATION SKILLS

It is generally accepted that effective communication requires appropriate knowledge, attitudes and skills (Faulkner, 1985; Macleod Clark and Webb, 1985). A similar requirement is necesssary for the teaching of communication skills. The survey therefore asked for feelings about knowledge and skills, and in addition contained a section on attitudes towards communication.

DNE's responses were correlated with their answers to the question 'How well prepared are tutors for the teaching of communication skills?' Tutors' responses were correlated with their answers to the question, 'In *your* opinion, how much training have you had for the teaching of communication skills?' These appeared to be central questions since it could be argued that if DNEs and tutors have positive attitudes, they would give priority to gaining the skills required and would be aware of limitations which require updating.

DNEs' attitudes

DNEs showed some positive correlations between their beliefs on the preparedness of tutors and their atttiudes to communication.

(1) Those who believed that communication skills are inherent in every human also believed that their tutors were well prepared to teach the subject ($p = 0.002$).
(2) DNEs who felt that their tutors were well prepared were more likely to believe that physical care should take precedent over emotional care ($p = 0.017$)
(3) The belief that tutors can happily use any teaching method was more likely to be held by those DNEs who were satisfied with their tutor preparation ($p = 0.009$).
(4) The belief that their tutors were well prepared was found to be linked to the belief that student nurses are well equipped to meet patients' emotional needs ($p = 0.001$).

There was a *negative* correlation between beliefs about tutor preparedness and the notion that communication is so important that it should be taught as a separate subject ($p = 0.005$). This may link with the beliefs that communication skills are inherent, which would certainly throw doubt on the need to teach it at all, let alone separately.

195

In terms of other attitude questions, there were no correlations. For example, although few schools had specialist teachers, 75% of DNEs agreed that communication should be taught by a specialist teacher. Similarly, although 53% of DNEs stated that communication was taught in every block, 98% agreed that the subject should be integrated into all blocks. These findings may suggest dissonance among DNEs between what actually happens in the curricula and what they perceive as the ideal.

Tutors' attitudes

There were no positive correlations between attitudes held and having been prepared for teaching communication skills in Scottish tutors, and only three correlations for tutors in the rest of Britain. Two of these were positive:

(1) Those who believed that communication skills are inherent in every human being were more likely to feel well prepared to teach communication skills ($p = 0.039$). In this, DNEs and tutors were in accord.
(2) Tutors who believed that they should be generalists were more likely to feel they were well prepared to teach communication skills than those who believed in specialism ($p = 0.022$)

There was a *negative* correlation between belief that it is possible to teach communication skills and the tutors' own preparedness ($p = 0.026$). This suggests, as with DNEs, that some tutors do not see communication as a subject to be taught.

As with DNEs the fact that there appears to be a difference between what happens in schools and colleges of nursing and what tutors believe personally gives potential for dissonance and for dissatisfaction with the current curricula. This state of affairs seems likely given the low number of tutors who felt they had been adequately prepared, and the high number who would like to attend a course.

Attitudes were also shown in individual comments at the end of the survey. One, from a DNE, sounded a little defensive: 'I have completed this questionnaire following discussion with all my staff. As you will see from it, we list communication as one of the priorities of our responsibilities as nurse educationists and all of us play an active part in ensuring that all people for whom we have an educational responsibility are made aware of the importance of communications.'

Tutors tended to comment more on the difficulties inherent in teaching the subject, for example, 'I wish that there was the time and finance to allow nurse teachers to further develop the skills required for communication teaching. There is also a great lack of information on how to actually teach communication. Much of it is done on a "hit or miss" basis'; or the more disillusioned tutor who commented 'I do not feel it is generally recognised by those responsible for nurse education that such things as communicative skills exist.'

This cry was echoed more positively by some tutors. One stated, 'It's lovely to see this type of information being requested — it suggests that at last people are beginning to look at this very important area', while another commented 'It [communication] is a very neglected area of nurse teaching.'

It is against this backdrop of attitudes and beliefs about communication in the curricula that the CINE project recruited two nurse teachers to act as research teachers in selected schools of nursing to test the effect of a planned programme of communication skills teaching.

THE CINE TEACHING INPUT

In recruiting tutors to the CINE project, there was the belief that, given appropriate training and periodic updating, any *committed* tutor could teach the planned programme of communication skills. The two tutors finally selected were different from each other on a number of points but they both shared a belief that communication was a vital part of the nursing curriculum. The tutor (South) had been a registered tutor for some time and had recently completed an MSc, and the tutor (North) was a social anthropologist and nurse who was working as a clinical teacher.

To share and update knowledge and skill, the teaching part of the project commenced with a four-day workshop in which the whole CINE team, which consisted of director, three associate directors, an evaluation officer and two research teachers were involved. This provided an opportunity to explore teaching methods, particularly experiential methods such as the use of warm-up games, role play, audio and audiovisual aids and feedback as a potential for learning.

This workshop was the first of a number of such opportunities, for the research teachers and the directors have continued to learn throughout the project.

When later the framework of the teaching sessions for learners was planned (Table 9.2) it was agreed that both teachers would cover the same content but that no attempt would be made to control teaching style. It was hoped that this would avoid the risk of 'cloning' while making the material, rather than the teacher's style, important.

The teaching input was evaluated using a quasi-experimental design incorporating pre-tests, post-tests and experimental and control groups. Four schools of nursing, two in the North of England and two in the South, were designated 'experimental' schools with two cohorts of students in each school receiving the teaching input and completing pre- and post-test evaluation measures. In addition, two schools of nursing, one in the North of England and one in the South, were designated 'control' schools with cohorts of students completing the pre- and post-tests measures while not receiving the CINE teaching input. A range of teaching methods were employed as shown in Table 9.3, but the emphasis was on an experiential approach, encouraging students to become actively involved in all sessions. The extent to which *teaching* staff in each school were involved with the teaching input varied considerably.

Some thought had to be given to the responsibilities inherent in taking a programme in to a school of nursing for a limited time. To avoid feelings of 'being used', staff at each experiential school were asked to nominate a 'link' tutor who would teach the research groups after the CINE data gathering was complete, and liaise with the CINE tutor during the project. Although there were some problems with this arrangement, most tutors involved took a very positive interest in the project and many were prepared to disclose feelings of inadequacy in relation to teaching communication skills. A full account of the researchers' experience in this area can be found in the Project Report (CINE, 1986).

During the project, one of the 'experimental' schools of nursing asked for a workshop for all their tutors to improve their experiential teaching skills, A residential weekend was arranged, but the content had to be changed to skills learning since the tutors realised, as a result of tape-recorded feedback sessions, that they did not have the skills that they were attempting to teach. A further follow-up workshop built on the skills training, and tutors explored different ways to teach the subject.

Table 9.2: Framework for communications skills input. Two introductory sessions, six skills sessions and as many sessions relating skills to practice as the individual programmes would allow

Session 1	*The place, importance and relevance of communication in nursing* An introduction to communication, human needs, health education, and the skills required for effective communication, including understanding self and others, attitudes, culture variables, etc.
Session 2	*Elements of communication* Detailed breakdown of verbal and non-verbal components of communication and skills needed for effective communication
Session 3	*Questioning skills* Obtaining information, assessing patients, types of questioning, purpose of each type, knowing appropriate use of each
Session 4	*Listening and attending skills* Listening habits, hearing, recognising cues, improving skill in listening, identifying cues and practising listening skills
Session 5	*Reinforcing and encouraging skills* Verbal and non-verbal encouragements, praise, valuing, repeating and reflecting
Session 6	*Information-giving skills* The purpose of giving information, facilitating and inhibiting the effective passage of information, factors related to each
Session 7	*Initiating and terminating interactions* Restrictions: time and environment, successful and unsuccessful openings and closings, factors leading to success, feelings and behaviour, review to date
Session 8	*Comfort and reassurance* Patient-centred behaviour, nurse-centred behaviour, purpose benefit, relationship formation, constructing barriers, research, health education, risk taking, self-disclosure
Session 9	*Combining micro-skills, nursing process* Assessing a patient and relatives' needs for communication, appropriate nursing behaviours, admissions of a patient, problem solving, goals
Session 10	*Communicating with other members of the health-care team* Authority, power and control, roles, attitudes, organisations, accountability, assertion, advocacy
Session 11	*Cancer and dying* Diagnosis, defence, denial, detachment, death, dying process, trust, empathy, sharing, identification, self-awareness
Session 12	*Preparing a patient for discharge* Health promotion, the nurse as a teacher, patient's rights, nurses' rights, education aims, alcoholism, heart disease, antenatal care, stoma patient discharge, smoking
Session 13	*Communicating with geriatric and stroke patients* Defining inhibiting factors, physiological failure of: sight, hearing, smell, taste, touch, movement. Frustration, denial, anger, rejection
Session 14	*Communicating with patients before and after surgery* Pre- and post-operative care, research findings, identifying fear, anxiety and recovery rate, reducing anxiety

Table 9.3: Teaching methods used in CINE sessions

Method	Example of use
1. Didactic	(a) Types of questions and appropriate use of questions (b) Theories (c) Research
2. Discussion (with or without stimulus material e.g. communication videos	To stimulate learning through attitude and experience sharing

3. Experiental	(a) Games: to encourage group cohesion
	(b) Exercises: to demonstrate the importance or effect of touch. To improve skills
	(c) Role play (with and without audio and video-recording and feedback)
	    (i) provides opportunity for self- and peer assessment;
	    (ii) provides feedback of skills development, e.g. questioning skills, listening skills.

EVALUATION OF THE EFFECT OF COMMUNICATION SKILLS TEACHING

The purpose of the evaluation process was to identify changes in students' perceptions, attitudes, skills and knowledge in relation to communication which could be attributed to the CINE input. Pre- and post-test assessments were undertaken by all students in experimental and control groups. Control and experimental groups were similar both in terms of demographic characteristics and in terms of academic achievement, previous experience and pre-test performance.

The pre- and post-test measures are outlined in Table 9.4, and covered written and behavioural aspects of communication skills. Post-test assessment showed that students in both groups gained improvements on their pre-test scores. However, those in the experimental groups demonstrated substantially greater increments in knowledge and skills than students in the control groups. These differences were particularly marked in terms of students' understanding and knowledge of the complexity of communication and in terms of the reactions and skills displayed when faced with more threatening or emotionally loaded situations. Full details of the methods used and data collected for the evaluation can be found in the project reports (CINE, 1986).

Table 9.4: Pre- and post-test evaluation

(a)	Personal
	(i) about self and background
	(ii) related to nursing
(b)	Case-history memory test: number of physical and psychological factors remembered
(c)	Attitudes
	(i) towards nursing
	(ii) towards communication
	(iii) towards communication skills teaching
(d)	Knowledge
	(i) about communication elements
	(ii) about communication skills
(e)	Skills/behaviour
	(i) video-recorded stimulus material and typewritten vignettes: coding based on students' written responses to patients' questions or statements
	(ii) video-recorded role plays of patient assessment interviews: coding based on verbal and non-verbal communication skills displayed, e.g. questioning, listening, encouraging, giving information

Interestingly the experimental groups emerged as feeling less confident of their ability to communicate well than the control group students. This finding may relate to their awareness of the complexities of communicating with patients and the opportunities they had for confronting their own and others' skills during role play and practice in the teaching session.

Some more descriptive data were collected from the project tutors and the students in the experimental groups concerning their perceptions of the communication skills teaching. Most of the students enjoyed the sessions and the teaching methods employed. For some it was their first experience of this approach and they welcomed the opportunity to contribute and participate. A small proportion of students (approximately 10%) did *not* enjoy the sessions, although most of these claimed to have learnt something from them.

The project tutors found that much of the teaching had to be done in smaller groups than those normally found in schools of nursing. They dealt with this by splitting their groups into two smaller groups of 12–14 students which meant, of course, doing twice the teaching. However, it was felt that tackling very large groups would have been totally unsatisfactory. In an ideal world, sessions involving communication skills practice would have a maximum of eight students to one tutor.

The project tutors found that it was advisable to delay the use of role play in the groups until a degree of group cohesion had developed and students had acquired some knowledge and confidence in clinical work. It was also found that videotapes and transcripts of real nurse-patient interactions were very useful for increasing students' awareness of communication problems and generating discussion in the absence of threat. Audiotape recordings were also found to be effective for giving students feedback on their own skills in the classroom and in the ward.

CINE PHASE II

In general it has to be accepted that this type of teaching is more demanding and stressful for tutors than conventional chalk-and-talk methods. This fact plus the findings from the project which illuminate the current lack of preparation received by tutors for this role have generated the momentum for a second phase of CINE. This second phase has been planned to explore the problems of helping nurse tutors acquire the knowledge and skills to teach communication skills. A great deal has been learned from the first phase of CINE but in some ways it has only been possible to raise awareness of the magnitude of the task and the difficulties inherent in trying to incorporate this essential material into the nursing curriculum.

The fact that awareness has been raised is confirmed by the response of tutor training establishments to the request that the CINE team be allowed to take over part of the curriculum to update tutor students' communication skills, and to teach experiential teaching methods. Only one college failed to reply to the request; the other four approached were keen to be involved. Of these, two were chosen at random to be involved throughout the academic year and the other two were offered workshops.

This stage of the project is currently under way. When the tutor students have completed their course, a random number will be followed up in their schools of nursing and monitored for their ability to put communication skills teaching into practice in their schools' curriculum, and to record the problems they encounter. The notion of peer support will also be monitored in that some students will return to schools which have had workshops for the rest of the teaching staff. These workshops are planned to raise awareness of the crucial importance of communication as part of the curriculum. There are no results to date except for a very positive response from the profession — in itself a crucial step forward.

CURRENT ISSUES

Since work on the project reported in this chapter commenced in 1980 the nursing profession has been subjected to many changes, most of which have served to illuminate the importance of communication skills to professional practice. We believe that there is now a general acceptance among nurses that communication skills need to be included in the basic nursing curriculum. However, there is less consensus about who, where and when it should be taught. As with all research, the CINE project is generating more questions than answers.

CONCLUSION

The CINE experiment has demonstrated that it *is* possible to integrate a substantial amount of communication skills teaching into programmes of nurse education and that students receiving this input demonstrate a significant increment in their knowledge, skills and, perhaps most importantly, their understanding and awareness of the complexities of communication. What we have also shown in that a great deal more teaching, practice and support are needed if student nurses are to develop their full potential as 'professional communicators'.

Moreover the profession has still to address the issues of updating and educating the vast numbers of practising nurses who have not had access to any formal communication skills training during either their education or their career. Society's expectations of nurses in the year 2000 will make even greater demands on their communication skills, as the health promotion and preventative care aspects of their role expand. It is unfair and unwise to fail to give trained nurses the preparation and support they will need to meet the challenge of changing roles.

The second phase of the CINE project is focusing on the issues of preparing tutors to take on a communicating skills teaching role. Again, to date, many new questions are being raised by the work. For example, is this an area which every tutor should teach? Certainly the methods employed in such teaching, such as role play, group work and exercises, should now become part of every teacher's repertoire, but it is less clear whether there is a need to develop a 'specialist' communication teaching role. Since communication is becoming even more central to all nursing activities, in hospital and the community, a strong case can perhaps be made for selecting a proportion of prospective nurse teachers on the basis of their commitment to communication skills teaching.

ACKNOWLEDGEMENTS

We are indebted to the Health Education Council for their generous support of this work. We are particularly grateful to Jane Randell for her foresight and encouragement, and to the CINE team members, Anne Tomlinson, Anne Williams, Brian Neeson and Christine Felsey.

REFERENCES

Ashworth, P. (1980) *Care to communicate*. Royal College of Nursing, London

Campbell, D.T. and Stanley, J.C. (1966) *Experimental and quasi-experimental designs for research*. Houghton Mifflin, Boston

CINE (1986) *Report of the Communication in Nursing Education Curriculum Development Project (Phase I)*. Health Education Council, London

Faulkner, A. (1980) The student nurse's role in giving information to patients, unpublished MLitt. thesis, University of Aberdeen

Faulkner, A. (1985). Getting it right. Counselling, in A. Faulkner and J. Macleod Clark (eds) *Communication nursing*. Bailliere Tindall, London

Faulkner, A. and Maguire P. (1984) Teaching assessment skills, in A. Faulkner (ed.) *Recent Advances in nursing: communication*. Churchill Livingstone, Edinburgh

James, D. (1975) Teaching in E. Raybould (ed.) *A Guide for teachers of nursing*. Blackwell Scientific Publications, London

Macleod Clark, J. (1982) Nurse–patient verbal interaction, unpublished PhD thesis, University of London

Macleod Clark, J. and Hunt, J. (eds) (1985) *Communication in patient care video teaching programmes*. Macmillan, London

Macleod Clark, J. and Webb, P. (1985) Health education — a basis for professional nursing practice. *Nurse Education Today, 5*, 210–14

Maguire, P. Tait, A. and Brooke, M. (1980) Mastectomy: a conspiracy of pretence. *Nursing Mirror, 150*, 17–19

Tomlinson, A., Macleod Clark, J. and Faulkner, A. (1984) Problems in experiential teaching. *Nursing Times, 80* (39), 45–7

10

Evaluation in Nursing Education

A.P. Gallego

INTRODUCTION

Evaluation has by tradition sustained an uneasy relationship with education. This may stem from some of the arguments that portray education exclusively as a process and unsuitable for scrutiny; therefore resolution of the issue of whether what is offered to the student is of any worth, or most important, how it could be improved, remains unattainable without evaluation.

In general education this picture is gradually changing. In the past 20 years great concern arising from individuals, schools and governments has resulted in the development of suitable approaches and methods that are more open to outside gaze. The information revealed has shown whether a system works and how it works. The past five years have seen the publication of Her Majesty's Inspectors' (HMI) reports on schools, which sometimes give rise to heated discussion. How would nursing education react to the publication of reports from the National Board for Nursing, Midwifery and Health Visiting resulting from visits by the Professional Education Officers?

There is another uneasy relationship which needs to be mentioned, that is the relationship between nursing education and nursing management. By tradition, the former has remained under the thumb of the latter. Evaluation could provide the route towards responsible autonomy. Nursing managers appear to have caught up more quickly than their educational counterparts with modern trends for increased evaluation; monitoring standards by measuring outcomes, identifying performance indicators or other such auditing systems have long been part of their language even if they are not yet operational throughout the country. It could be argued that by not asking nurse teachers to give an account of their performance, nurse managers keep education under control and in a subservient position. This point will be developed later in the chapter.

The chapter will address itself to the meanings and interpretations of the word 'evaluation'; possible models for evaluation will be presented; and instances of internal and external school evaluation and the processes involved in both will be discussed. Finally the implications for nursing education will be emphasised.

LEVELS OF EVALUATION

Evaluation involves the systematic collection of information for the purpose of decision making. It can take place at different levels. Ideally it should start with individuals looking at their own performance with the purpose of monitoring the development and thereby improving the outcome. *Self-evaluation* is eclectic and makes use of different perspectives such as: results from an appraisal, curriculum vitae, test results, feedback from 'the client', and sickness/absence ratios. I will refer to the next level as *peer evaluation*. This is a feature of a professional group where relationships are in principle collegial rather than hierarchical. The appraisal system within the National Health Service was possibly based on this concept, but as nursing occurs mainly within a bureaucratic system and is hierarchical in nature, it has not developed as either an informal or a formal system. The next level, *institutional evaluation*, is the evaluation carried out by an institution such as the school, the hospital, a ward or a unit. Finally there is a *central evaluation*: the evaluation carried out by the National Board, the DHSS, and the health district.

In the first three levels, control over the information gathered should remain theoretically with the individual or the unit: internal evaluation. It should be up to the individual or group to decide what knowledge is to be used and who is to have access to it. But if we think back to the purpose of evaluation, rarely can decisions be made in isolation; the decisions taken by one person or unit usually affect other people and other units who then become entitled to know. Indeed, they may demand to know.

Centrally based evaluation (or external evaluation) implies some form of external control which in turn presupposes public accounting of decisions that may be taken.

INTERPRETATIONS OF THE WORD 'EVALUATION'

Evaluation means different things to different people. In Table 10.1 I have gathered some of the most common interpretations of the word. Mainly these fall into two categories, each conferring different values to the term and which represent contrasting styles of evaluation: measurement vs judgement; quantitative vs qualitative. These categories arise from the value accorded to the information that needs to be gathered.

Table 10.1: Interpretations of the word 'evaluation'

Quantitative	versus	Qualitative
Measurement		*Judgement*
Monitoring of standards		Value
Measure of efficiency		Quality assurance
Measure of outcomes/objectives		
Auditing		
Cost-effectiveness		Questions about worth
Performance indicators		Appraisal
Evaluation for accountability		Evaluation for professional development

Table 10.2 summarises the main differences between the two styles. The subheadings: theoretical approach, methodology, sources of data, etc. loosely describe the evaluation process, which in turn closely mirrors the research process. In spite of their differing purposes these two processes are similar.

In general education, a balanced approach has been advocated by such authors as Lawton (1978), Eisner (1978) and McCormick and James (1983). Walker (1977) is concerned with the relationship between qualitative evaluation and the desire to provide a more complex basis for decision-making. He argues that evaluators should be more aware of the political contexts within which their studies are located. He sees useful evaluation reports as having a dual commitment:

(a) to the understanding of the complexity of social actions; and
(b) to be useful for those acting in complex situations.

In nursing education a different picture seems to emerge. Carpenter (1978) describes the schism in nursing between what he

207

Table 10.2: Two contrasting (or complementary) styles of evaluation

Quantitative	Qualitative
(1) *Terminology*	
Scientific	Ethnographic
Product	Process
Classical/traditional 'objectives'	Illuminative (Parlett and Hamilton, 1972)
	Holistic (Macdonald, 1974)
(2) *Theoretical approach*	
Specific	'Grounded'; relates to setting
Explicit	Shaped by the setting
Hypothesis testing	
Deductive	Inductive
(3) *Methodology*	
Sampling: adequate, random	Based in setting
	Culture specific
Objective criteria	Beyond quantification
	Controlled subjectivity
Behaviour outcome	Behaviour: cue to understanding
Validity/reliability	Evaluator — the instrument
(4) *Sources of data*	
Verbal	Verbal/non-verbal
Behavioural	Observation: participant/ non-participant
Records	Diaries
Statistical	Accounts
(5) *Evaluator's approach*	
Clear role: evaluator/researcher	Sensitive to entry and role
Concerned with control	Identification
Concerned with elimination of error	Development of trust leading to shared information
(6) *Skills*	
Scientific, numerate	Awareness
Research design	Empathy
Selected objectivity	Controlled objectivity
Representative sample	—
Non-involvement	Participant
(7) *Conclusions, report*	
Asocial	Case study; quick feedback
Generalisable	Accepts uniqueness
Reproducible	
Publishable	Publication needs to be negotiated
Anonymity	Confidentiality

called 'managerialists' and 'professionalists'. The managerialists are more concerned with the organisational form of the service than with its nature. They identify with managerial reference groups and therefore would subscribe to those values that are concerned with product, cost-effectiveness and output. The professionalists have identified with bedside nursing and its ideologies which emphasise the nature of the service provided and the quality of care.

Teachers of nursing do not appear to have developed an occupational strategy congruent with their role, by, for example, pursuing academic excellence, and developing an academic identity. As a group they seem split, a condition that is perhaps helped by the organisational structure in which they work, which encourages the director of nursing education and senior tutor grade to become 'managerialists'. Nevertheless, it may be true to say that most teachers of nursing are more in sympathy with the values of the 'professionalists'. This may explain the apparent gap/misunderstanding which sometimes seems to exist between nurse teachers and nurse managers. Whereas the former may be thinking in terms of the 'worth of education', the latter are more concerned with its cost-effectiveness. There is no reason why both approaches could not complement one another, my argument being that if nursing education is to survive, it needs to develop evaluation models which illuminate both the worth and cost-effectiveness of education.

MODELS FOR EVALUATION

Traditionally evaluation models have been broadly divided under the categories of quantitative/qualitative already mentioned. Table 10.3 summarises their main characteristics.

I would now like to consider evaluation in relation to two parameters: knowledge and control. The first parameter exemplifies many of the assumptions inherent in the conflict between quantitative and qualitative models for evaluation. Definitions of knowledge can be placed on a continuum ranging from knowledge that is considered objective, scientific and positivist in nature to knowledge that is perceived as subjective, relativistic and ethnographic. The second parameter, the issue of control, is also an important one in relation to evaluation. Macdonald (1974) classified evaluation studies into three ideal types according to who controls the pursuit of new knowledge and who has access to it. Control could be exercised by the evaluator (autocratic) or the group or unit

Table 10.3: Main characteristics of quantitative and qualitative models for evaluation

Quantitative	*Qualitative*
Favours a hypothetico-deductive approach	Favours a problem-solving inductive approach or grounded theory
Relies on quantitative methodology	Involves qualitative methods of research
At its most basic level this model would involve: pre-test → teaching programme →post-test	Compared with quantitative models, they are more extensive and complex as they are not merely restricted to test data
It emphasises product-efficiency criteria, i.e. wastage rates, examination results, student-teacher ratios	It emphasises criteria that portray the process and the context where it all happens. Accurate portrayal and sensitive interpretation are stressed. The evaluation builds up a continuous record of events, transactions, informal remarks documenting a broad spectrum of phenomena, judgements and responses, adding interpretive comments
Favoured by the objectives model of curriculum development which perceives evaluation as an examination of whether derived objectives — expressed in behavioural terms — are or are not attained	Favoured by the process model of curriculum development which perceives evaluation as reflecting: 'The process of teaching, learning and schooling, the outcomes we could reasonably expect from such transactions and the strengths and weaknesses of educational provision' (Simons, 1980a)
Evaluation in this context is very much a measure of efficiency	Evaluation is seen primarily as a tool to enhance the professional development of teachers and the personal growth of students

from whom the information is gathered (democratic) or by the organisation who commissioned the study (bureaucratic). Control can also be *implicit* such as the control exercised by the teacher and the expert, or *explicit* as in rules and regulations and policy statements issued by the organisation.

Evaluation can then be classified according to its relation with these two parameters, and a structural map can be developed resulting in four different models: managerial, professional, democratic and participative. Underlying each model there are distinct institutional, occupational and ideological perspectives.

Figure 10.1 shows the relations between these four models and their respective styles. In Figure 10.2 the relations between the different methods of evaluation used under each of the models are illustrated.

Two points need to be made. First, theoretical models are made up of typical characteristics of the general category or issue that they represent and as such are helpful to guide, describe and analyse a particular situation but in practice they rarely exist in their pure form because they contain many stereotypes. Secondly there is a considerable degree of overlap between the four models, so, in practice, elements of the four will be present to a greater or lesser degree in any school of nursing that is engaged in evaluation. Nevertheless, the conceptual maps offered may be useful to analyse some of the present dilemmas impinging on evaluation in nursing education.

Figure 10.1: Models of evaluation

	Objective Quantitative	
Professional Autocratic, the teacher: in authority and an authority; Academic excellence *Education a professional concern*	*Managerial* Bureaucratic, output, productivity measurement, cost *Cost-effectiveness; value for money*	
Individual Implicit		
		Collective Explicit
Democratic Individualised education, learner participation, individual interests *Education a shared concern*	*Participative* Institutional context, cultural and political issues. Participants and context share power *Education an activity influenced by its context*	
	Subjective Qualitative	

Figure 10.2: Methods used under different models of evaluation

	Objective Quantitative
Professional	*Managerial*
— Examination results	— Recruitment and selection procedures
— Measurable objectives	— Examination results
— Students' evaluation of course	— Wastage rates
	— Employment profiles
Q. Were the objectives of the course achieved?	Q. Is the school training people who can provide for the needs of the institution and who will later fit the organisation?

Individual
Implicit

Collective
Explicit

Democratic	*Participative*
— Selection procedures	— Analysis of archives
— Personal interviews	— Context of school
— Students' evaluation	i) environment
— Course materials	ii) organisational structure
	— Profiles of teachers
	— Biographies of participants
Q. How is the course meeting your needs? Is it what you expected it to be?	Q. Within the context of the institution, how do teachers and students see their role and interact with the system?

Subjective
Qualitative

PRESENT DILEMMAS IN EVALUATING NURSING EDUCATION

At the present time the struggle between nursing managers and nurse teachers keeps evaluation firmly within the managerial and professional models.

In nursing, the management structure is at present more powerful. This is reflected in the emphasis placed on service needs at the expense of educational requirements. The English National Board (ENB) policies promote an objectives model of curriculum by specifying nursing competencies in behavioural terms, which in turn would favour an objectives model of evaluation (professional model). There has also been a general move towards a process model of education but particularly so in psychiatric nurse education, encouraged by the 1982 Mental Nurse Training Syllabus.

The introduction of the nursing process, a humanistic approach to patient/client care which centres around the needs of the individual, could help towards a move to the democratic model, provided it is not adopted as a strategy towards professionalisation (Dickinson, 1982). Davis (1983) discussed the application of the nursing process to the process model of education with particular reference to nurse training. This model would cater for individual learner needs and would encourage a shift towards the democratic and participative models of evaluation.

I would now like to present an example of evaluation which has features of the four models. It concentrates on evaluating the school, and although it may not be a practical scheme in its entirety, there may be elements of it that could be adapted for individual use.

EVALUATING THE SCHOOL: A CASE STUDY

The purpose of the study

The purpose of the study was to evaluate the existing theoretical curriculum of a three-year basic nurse training programme in a school of nursing based in a London teaching hospital by focusing on one team of teachers concerned with SRN training and the effect upon two sets of students. A system of two-week blocks had been introduced as an intermediate step towards a modular system of training. The system it replaced consisted of four-week blocks which occurred roughly once a year.

A case-study approach was adopted in which the characteristics of an individual unit — in this case a school — were observed. Cohen and Manion (1980) maintained that the purpose of such observation is to probe deeply and to analyse the unit intensively with a view to establishing generalisations about the wider population to which the unit belongs. Readers, though, must weigh carefully the situation presented to them and decide which aspects are applicable in their particular case.

The case-study approach is an antithesis to the statistical, quantitative style and has been used extensively in anthropology, sociology, education, medicine and psychiatry. The aim of the report was to make its content relevant to the audience for whom it was particularly intended: the staff of the school under study. A wide range of techniques were employed in the collection and analysis of both qualitative and quantitative data, but methodologically observation remained the pivot throughout the study.

Ethical issues

The case study approach raises important ethical issues which are applicable to the process of evaluation as a whole. I would like to concentrate on two of these issues: anonymity and the right of every individual to privacy.

The evaluator should operate as if both anonymity and privacy are likely to be violated. Therefore the evaluator must be not only sensitive to the situation she is reporting but must also share an explicit code of conduct with those who are under investigation. This explicit code of conduct could take the form of a contract which is periodically negotiated and which contains the following features:

(1) Informed consent. The evaluator must satisfy herself that the group/unit involved fully understands the aims of the exercise and the kinds of knowledge wanted. Several authors, such as Pring (1984) and Simons (1977), maintain that as it is practically impossible to anticipate all the information required, this provides a continuing opportunity to renegotiate the terms of contract.
(2) The issues of who controls the information gained and who has access to it should be discussed at the initial stages and certainly before gathering data.
(3) The evaluator should show throughout the process her 'papers': the data collected (or selected) and the interpretation of the data.
(4) The evaluator throughout should be open to cross-examination by the group.
(5) The evaluator is obliged to incorporate into her findings the reply, if any, of those into whom research was carried out.
(6) The 'right to know' could collide with some of the fundamental principles underlying the respect for another person's theory. Therefore the evaluator should be particularly aware of such issues as: not betraying trust and confidence, trying not to hurt, and keeping promises.

214

As part of the process of evaluation there is a question of trust and mutual respect which a contract alone cannot capture but which the evaluator must be constantly aware of and which must form part and parcel of her responsibilities.

Data gathered

For the sake of clarity I have organised this section under four headings: profile of the school; profile of the institution (the combination of school and hospital); profile of the students; and profile of the teachers. Profiling entails giving an outline, a schematic description, of the main features of an institution or set of individuals. The profile includes both quantitative and qualitative 'measures'. A multi-faceted approach was adopted, and the methods used were characteristic of the four models of evaluation mentioned in Figure 10.1.

Profile of the school

This was drawn from:

(1) A study of archives, with particular reference to:

(a) The *League News*. In the late 1890s the trained nurses at this institution formed a League and published a journal. This provided a very good record of training, of life at the hospital and of the characteristics of the nurse at the institution.
(b) a notebook of a student nurse in the 1890s;
(c) annual reports of the senior tutor in charge of the school to matron;
(d) school programmes, with particular reference to the General Nursing Council (GNC) syllabuses and their impact on the programmes produced.

The archives were studied to show the approach adopted to the development of the curriculum since 1877 which was when the institution opened a school of nursing.
(2) A study of the school geographical environments.
(3) A study of the organisational structure in terms of decision-making and communication channels.

Profile of the institution

A profile of the institution was included because in nursing education we have two curricula: the practical and the theoretical, and
students spend up to 80% of their training in the clinical situation.
The profile was drawn from a study of archives with particular
reference to policy statements, the *League News*, and the records of
prominent nurses (including textbooks written by them) who had
played an important role in the historical development of the
institution.

The aim of the study was to capture the ethos of the institution
and its underlying ideological system as this is a major influence on
the hidden curriculum and on the trained nurse who will be the
guardian and transmitter of the values and mores of the institution
to future generations of nurses. Illuminative evaluators call it 'the
learning milieu' (Parlett and Hamilton, 1972). Sociologists refer to
'culture', meaning the shared norms, common values, understand-
ings and agreements that bind together those within the institution
(Musgrove, 1973). Durrell's poetic term 'spirit of place' is also a
good description (1969). Both accounts involving the school and the
institution were cross-checked with several colleagues and amended
to incorporate their perceptions.

Profile of the students

The convenience sample constituted two sets of students numbering
48 and 44 respectively ($N=92$). Quantitative data were gathered
including age, educational qualifications, parents' occupations, and
work experience. The recruitment, selection and admission procedures were examined, including information given to prospective
candidates and interviewing criteria, among others. The success rate
was quantitatively analysed. This included: end of block results, end
of first-year examination results, practical assessment results, ward
reports and final state and hospital examination results. Wastage rate
was also included. Qualitative data were obtained from the students'
personal-tutor records. Closed-circuit television recordings of group
discussions in different classes with different teachers were also used
and cross-checked with sociograms constructed during 'management
games'. Personal recollections were checked against student records
and colleagues who were members of the teaching team. Every set
elected a leader, and the different leadership styles were also
examined.

Students' evaluation of their course and tutors involved the analysis of 14 block evaluation forms (seven for each set of students).

These evaluations were designed as structured questionnaires, which became unstructured in the third year of training (Gallego, 1983). It was decided not to interview students as a great deal of data had been gathered from them.

Profile of the teachers

This group included six teachers who had been members of the teaching team directly responsible for the two sets of students. The teachers were asked to draw their own profiles and were given three headings as guidelines: brief professional background, personality characteristics, and personal beliefs. Three preferred to be interviewed rather than write their own statement. Notes were taken during the interviews, which when written in full were first checked with the interviewee. The subject then selected a colleague whose function it was to validate whether the profile drawn reflected her own perception of that individual. Therefore for each teacher profile there were three people involved. Of all the teachers approached, none objected, but this was without any doubt the hardest of all procedures for both the evaluator and the 'subjects'.

The director of nurse education and two other colleagues (not part of the teaching team) were interviewed and a semi-structured schedule used around the question: 'What do you think of the present two-week block system?' Each interview when transcribed was cross-checked with the interviewee.

Findings

The findings will be presented for three chronological periods: 1877–1960, 1960–1970, and 1970–1979.

1877–1960

The origins of the institution were very ancient and the history of nursing there had clearly traceable religious roots. The school of nursing was opened in 1877. Training lasted for one year and was entirely practical with a few evening lectures by doctors who also demonstrated procedures. Other personnel like the 'bathman' were responsible for showing the 'probationers' special tasks. Later the training was increased to three years and in 1906 to four years, remaining so until the 1970s. Probationers in the beginning worked a 96-hour week. By the 1920s they were doing a 56-hour week, and conditions of service had generally improved. Nurse training developed from the occasional lecture/demonstration during off-duty hours to a pattern of prescribed evening or early morning sessions.

In 1925 the preliminary training school (PTS) was opened away from the main hospital, as was the practice in other establishments, and the first sister tutor was appointed. The probationers spent the first 12 weeks of their course mostly in the classroom within a fairly secluded environment which helped to create a feeling of set identity and to socialise the nurse into the hospital culture (Dodd, 1973). At the end of the first year there was an examination. The material for the second and third year which had been determined by the GNC 1923 syllabus was covered following the pattern of evening or early morning lectures.

All institutions had to design their training programmes to fit in with the GNC syllabuses. Since its inception, the GNC has published five: 1923, 1952, 1962, 1969 and 1977, and accordingly changes in the pattern of training of this institution reflected each new syllabus.

During the 1950s a 'study days' system was introduced, and in 1954 (as the result of the GNC 1952 syllabus) the theoretical component of the programme was enlarged and three four-week blocks coinciding roughly with the students' first, second and third year of training were introduced. This pattern of long blocks of theory, mostly medically orientated, persisted until 1976.

The institution was never short of applicants, and it produced through role-modelling and socialisation a well defined nurse:

A well mannered, refined Anglo-Saxon woman with deep religious convictions, keen eyed, brisk of movement, incisive of speech. High esteem is placed on conformity to the role resulting in disciplined nurses with a strong sense of comradeship and unity, very proud of their hospital and confident of their own worth, their motto throughout the years of service has been 'The patient comes first'. (A.P. Gallego, 1980)

Candidates were selected to suit the role image. Recruitment was mainly by word of mouth and family tradition, and the educational and social background of the trainees remained fairly static throughout the years. Many nurses once trained remained in the parent hospital. There was a well defined system for appointing trained staff to senior positions, and most of these were occupied by nurses trained by the institution.

The philosophy of the institution was covertly expressed through strong ideas of service: to the patient and to the doctor (the nurse was seen as the doctor's helper). Nursing was seen as a practice discipline, and, as such, great emphasis was placed on demonstrations and practical skills.

Nursing was seen clearly as a vocation, a 'calling'. The doctors were in control, but sister was 'in charge' of ward and patient and knew best what was good for both. The hidden curriculum transmitted and maintained this ideology and would modify or block those influences that threatened the ethos of the institution (Dodd, 1973; Gallego, 1983). Both the theoretical and the practical curriculum were product-orientated, and evaluation was based solely on examination and test results.

1960–1970

At the end of the 1960s, this institution, which up till then had remained fairly impervious to outside influences, was faced with 'Salmonisation' (Report of the Committee on Senior Nursing Staff, 1966 — commonly known as the Salmon report), when people not trained in the institution were appointed to senior positions.

The school was also faced with change: the introductory course came to the hospital and this move allowed the students easier access to the patients, which had implications for the planning of their programme. The school increased the teaching time to 25 weeks, and in 1968 the first integrated degree course started, thus extending the range of candidates; a school for pupil nurses was opened in 1970 which allowed girls of lower academic ability but interested in bedside nursing to train for the Roll at this teaching hospital.

Change threatens security. All institutions tend towards conservatism, and in the face of change they fight to preserve the stable state: what Schon (1971) identified as 'dynamic conservatism'. This institution was no exception.

During this period, Dodd used the institution in her PhD thesis, which was completed in 1973. In her study she was concerned with exploring the hospital context as a learning environment for nurses in training. She interviewed first- and third-year nurses to try to elucidate how these girls experienced the training process. She also interviewed fourth-year nurses, ward sisters, tutors and doctors. The report depicted an institution undergoing change in spite of itself; there was low morale and dissatisfaction was felt among the nursing staff.

219

From the data, Dodd identified certain trends:

(1) Students found a low correlation between the ideal situation (as taught in the school) and the real situation (as experienced in the clinical area).

(2) The tutor was perceived as a 'teacher of ideal nursing for examination purposes'. The learner saw the role of the school as relevant to examinations only. It was thought that the knowledge offered by the school was not related to the knowledge needed for doing the job of nursing. Even the practical assessments (which are ward-based practical examinations and an integral part of the total assessment for registration) were seen as a form of confrontation between the carrier of the ideal and the real; the tutors were seen as not fitting into the clinical context for two main reasons:

(a) their commitment to the ideal made them unfit for the clinical teaching role and would only cause clinical chaos;

(b) their presence would not be appreciated by sister, who would perceive the tutor as threatening (as well as disruptive).

(3) Students were also critical of the teaching programme: the lack of coherence; the passive teaching methods employed; the low teaching standards (seen particularly by respondents with A levels) and the excessive amount of control and discipline.

At the time, all tutors taught in every block and met every set of students. Each tutor was allocated a number of students from different sets for academic follow-up, counselling and individual tuition if necessary. Most tutors taught their specialist subject, but this system did not suit every tutor. Some felt that nursing was moving towards a more generalist curriculum, and that teaching by principles was more important than specific procedures or local methods. As many tutors were involved in the theoretical training of students, proper co-ordination of the learning experience was problematic. Another major source of dissatisfaction was the fact that although all tutors met all sets, a tutor would know a very small number of students in a particular set.

Dodd arrived at the unhappy conclusion that 'Any caring institution offering a training programme which fails to take into account the perspectives of trainees and clients cannot be called educational.'

She also determined in her study that the hospital used a medical model and that nurses could not solve their problems and change under this model.

The thesis could be considered an evaluation of the existing system carried out by an outside evaluator. It certainly served as a baseline study for me from which to evaluate developments in the subsequent ten years. However, Dodd's thesis was totally ignored by the institution, a classical example of the 'rejection syndrome' described by Rapoport in 1970. Dodd produced a report shortly after collecting her data in which she summarised the results and presented some tentative findings. No recollection of such a document was elicited, except from the director of nursing education. The institution did not attempt an evaluation of its own. It appeared as if the study had never taken place.

1970–1979

In the early 1970s, partly as the result of Salmon and partly due to the Report of the Committee on Nursing (1972 — commonly known as the Briggs report), the school altered its staff deployment and pattern of training.

Salmon meant, for the school staff, job descriptions, formalised areas of responsibility and lines of control. The staff was reorganised into teaching teams, each team originally consisted of three members, one senior tutor, one tutor and a clinical teacher. A team was responsible for the planning of blocks, the academic follow-up and counselling, and the writing of student reports at the end of each block. Later, the pattern of training changed, indicating a move towards a modular system of training. The blocks became shorter and occurred more frequently through the three-year training. Nine two-week blocks, together with secondments to psychiatry, geriatrics, nursing community care and obstetric nursing, mostly outside the parent hospital, were offered to the students.

The institution was faced with even greater change as the result of the 1974 NHS reorganisation, which meant acquiring district responsibilities. The institution was forced to 'open up'. The learners no longer trained at the parent hospital only, but also divided their training between two other hospitals within the district, which represented different demographic and ideological stances: the encounter with different ethnic groups exhibiting different needs and problems; the sharing of funds; the increased demand for accountability with the corresponding loss of autonomy, power and prestige; a different institutional ethos with other traditions; and hospitals which may have perceived the parent hospital as wanting to take over. These attitudes were transmitted to the students who went to the different hospitals to gain clinical experience, and gave rise to conflict and stress.

Shortly afterwards, the school became a district school with approximately 1000 students. It prepared six intakes a year of 50 students each for SRN training; it also trained for the Roll, had an integrated degree course in conjunction with a local university by which the students after four years could obtain an SRN certificate and a social sciences degree, and a number of post-basic courses.

The school moved into a purpose-built modern building situated in the grounds of the parent hospital. The organisational structure consisted of one director of nursing education (DNE), two assistant directors (ADNE) and nine teaching teams. Six teams were concerned with SRN training, and functioned fairly autonomously. The leadership of the school was along hierarchical lines, with information being passed downwards mostly from DNE to senior tutor and tutor. The relationships between the teams were mostly informal, and the learners socialised mainly with members of their own set. The curriculum operating in the school could be described as teacher-centred, with a predominance of formal methods of teaching and a fairly rigid timetable divided into hourly periods with approximately two study periods during a two-week block. The overall philosophy transmitted via the hidden curriculum remained unchanged. So did the selection procedures.

The students and teachers

Although the aim of the case study was to focus on the role of the team concerned with SRN training and its effect upon two sets of students, interestingly and unexpectedly the institutional context became an increasingly important character as the story unfolded until it nearly took over. I will now return to the students (identified as sets 76 and 77) and their teachers by presenting their profiles.

Profile of sets 76 and 77

Both sets were representative of other sets in the school and indeed they were also very similar to Dodd's findings in the 1970s. The information is summarised in Table 10.4 (for further information see Gallego, 1983).

Profile of the teachers

Set 76 changed leader twice, set 77 three times during their training. The first leader was possibly more autocratic and formal in her

Table 10.4: Profile of sets 76 and 77 ($n = 92$)

Recruitment	Mainly by word of mouth and family tradition
Age distribution	Range: 18–22 years

Age	%
18	11
19	59
20	20
21	5
22	5

	No. of O and A levels	%
Educational qualifications	5 O	5
	6 O or more	12
	1–4 A	83

	Social class	%
Student's social background according to parents' stated occupation	I–II	83
	III	17

Ethnic origin	All came from UK; one student Indian
Gender	All female
Status	None married when training commenced

Examination results*	Set 76	Set 77
	Final State 90%	85%
	First year 100%	88%

Both groups very similar on ward reports and practical assessments. Set 77 had slightly higher percentage block marks overall throughout their training. Statistically not significant

Wastage rate	Set 76	Set 77
	8%	16%

School average: 13–15%

Profiles of the sets (from sociograms, CCTV, etc.)

Set 76: very united; had three leaders: administrative, spokesman, recreation; no obvious cliques; a group who functioned well as a team and who produced their best work under group conditions by pooling resources

Set 77: group divided into cliques; very competitive; group work unpredictable; some individual performances outstanding

* School average: 92–95%

relationships with the students than the other two leaders that followed her. Her major characteristic was that she was a change agent and encouraging to colleagues to develop their new ideas further. The second leader could be described as a democrat, but a great believer that people should be taught how to exercise their democratic rights responsibly. She was very keen on experiential methods of learning and small group work. This tradition was continued by the third leader who was more *laissez-faire* and who favoured and practised a student-centred and humanistic approach to learning.

From the data collected it became apparent that the way the block content was interpreted and organised reflected the ideology of the team leader. Also certain team combinations were more successful than others in presenting a common ideology.

The students' evaluation of their course and teachers

Bearing in mind that the evaluator analysed summaries of 14 block evaluations (seven for each set) and four *complete* block evaluation questionnaires from set 76 and two complete ones from set 77, only a very brief summary can be presented here.

The aims of evaluating courses were explained to the students during the introductory course, and the questionnaire was introduced at some length to encourage the students to assess their course seriously and to be positively critical. The exercise was seen as one promoting personal growth and experimentally showing the students — and teachers — how to evaluate other facets of their work.

The students evaluated not only content but also their lecturers; they took an interest in teaching methods and new schemes; they provided the team with useful suggestions which were passed on to other teams and sometimes taken up by the whole school; changes were effected as the direct result of students' suggestions; other aspects of their training also appeared in the comments, such as on clinical teaching, on the clinical setting, on students' welfare, and on allocation. The comments also depicted the nature of the student-teacher relationship. The students seemed to identify with the team tutors and this gave both students and teachers a sense of belonging. There was a dialogue, a process of negotiation and debate, which on occasions caused the tutors and the students strain, but which in most instances they were able to resolve satisfactorily for both parties.

Discussion

In 1979 the school underwent a major curriculum review and produced a theoretical curriculum which had the following features:
— it demonstrated a shift from a medical model to a nursing model of care;
— the curriculum became integrated around nursing themes;
— there was a slight shift from biological to social sciences;
— there was a shift from teacher-centredness to student-centredness.

Findings of the case study

The case study is a study of conflict. At one level, if we describe power in terms of bureaucracy, autocracy and democracy, the case study examines how the student of this institution pays allegiance to these three powers, and experiences very conflicting messages which create role conflict.

I would not nurse in an establishment as large and hierarchical as P again.

I feel it's rather sad that the challenge and trauma has been caused by staff — not patients — . . . It hasn't been easy to maintain one's self-esteem and individuality — it can be knocked out easily in a bureaucratic system but this doesn't lead to happy, well-balanced nurses or good nursing care . . . By using our personalities and interests, greater benefit could have been gained — we are all intelligent and by using some of this personal insight in the clinical situation new ideas and practice could be established, furthering nursing as a whole. I have appreciated the type of education in school, i.e. evaluation forms, guided studies, etc. This is contradictory to how things work in practice but I work better in a more relaxed environment.

Third-year student nurse

At another level the conflict also appears to be one of dissonance between the hospital and the school with regard to the nursing model taught in one and practised in another and the model of education and the methods used to transmit it. Dodd (1973), Bendall (1975) and Kramer (1974) have documented well the ideal-reality conflict. Kramer believed that in order for growth to occur conflict must be present, but it *must be managed constructively*. Referring back to the

225

case study, the 1979 changes could have been the end product of previous conflict. Nurses must be prepared to manage conflict so that personal growth can take place. These students, who will provide the future trained staff of the institution, must be able to challenge the institutional context and help and participate in the change and growth of their work environment.

This study has raised various issues. I would like to leave the reader with some questions:

— Does your institution take into account the perspectives of trainees and clients?
— Do you in the school use the students as agents of change?
— Are you in the school prepared to evaluate yourselves: to evaluate your own performance honestly and without outside pressures?

SCHOOL SELF-EVALUATION: AN INTERNAL PROCESS

The concept of the self-evaluative school has a strong appeal, especially if done at first on a small scale using simple methods with perhaps an experienced outside evaluator to act in a consultative capacity.

Simons (1980b) pointed out that much of the information that would form the data base is already there in the school in the form of examination results, timetables, minutes of teacher meetings, policy documents, and the state and content of noticeboards. To these the reports of interviews, observation, tape recordings and other material relevant to the chosen issue could be added. The difficulty lies in compiling this in a form that is easy to assimilate and discuss. Perhaps the first self-evaluative exercise should focus on a specified issue, not too complex, so that the scope of the study is limited, the questions can be easily framed and a focus on personalities can be avoided.

The case study that has been presented is complex but its initial purpose, to review the curriculum, was in itself very broad. At the beginning, small-scale, simple self-evaluating exercises may serve as a base for a more ambitious activity in the future. The important aspect is to break new ground and plant the seed.

Helen Simons argues for school-process self-evaluation — internally managed — on the basis that it will enhance the professional image and practice of teachers and schools. She relates this to the current accountability debate and warns schools against responding to outside pressure by producing whatever is required of them 'without themselves using the data for review of the professional practice of the school' (Simons, 1980a).

In the next section some of the issues involved in centrally based evaluation will be explained by focusing on how courses are approved in higher education and schools of nursing.

THE POLITICS OF EVALUATION

Current issues

The central political argument surrounding evaluation is that of autonomy versus accountability. Can a compromise be reached, or are the positions so entrenched that they become mutually exclusive? Evaluation discloses information about the system under study. Under the principle that knowledge is power, this disclosure could make the system more vulnerable. Lawton (1978) discussed this issue in relation to general education and maintained that the request from central government for greater accountability would eventually mean greater central control and consequently less autonomy for general education.

I would like to compare levels of control in higher education and nursing education within schools of nursing by focusing on the procedures involved for the approval of basic nursing courses. It can be argued that this is an aspect where the evaluation process surfaces; it becomes public and therefore fully visible and explicit. A course is submitted, it is centrally reviewed (evaluated); if the course is thought good it is approved and if not it is rejected.

In higher education, evaluation is well established particularly within polytechnics. Universities function somewhat independently, each university having its own validating body and procedures. Within polytechnics and other higher education institutions, the Council for National Academic Awards (CNAA) is responsible for the approval of courses and plays an important role within a well established procedure. It issues guidelines for course planning which are fairly non-specific and allow for a great deal of flexibility. The CNAA is composed of specialist panels which provide a combination of expert advice and peer evaluation. The course planning group (CPG) can ask for such advice at any stage of the development of the submission or course document.

According to Becher and Maclure (1978) the main features of the

CNAA's validation process are:

(1) it is a regular and formal procedure;
(2) it is essentially peer evaluation;
(3) it involves a thorough evaluation.

Course approval in higher education

The stages involved in course approval are shown in Figure 10.3. The resource statement is similar to the ENB's (1985) 'application for approval in principle' document. The resource statement has first to be approved internally by the appropriate polytechnic committee, which looks at whether there is a need for such a course, whether there are resources available and whether the course fits into the general strategy of the institution. External approval is then sought from the Department of Education and Science (DES), the Regional Advisory Committee (RAC) and, for nursing courses that are statutory, the ENB. Once approval in principle has been obtained, the CPG develops a course submission along the guidelines provided by the CNAA.

Once the submission has been completed, many institutions mount an internal vetting procedure which reflects the CNAA vetting exercise. The aim of this procedure is for the panel to evaluate all aspects of the proposed course, and to look for its strengths and weaknesses with the intention of reinforcing the former and eliminating the latter. The internal vetting not only serves as a trial run but also helps the CPG to rehearse and plan the defence of the course and the arguments that they will use to an outside panel.

An internal vetting panel consists of members of the institution's top management (the director, or assistant director); and a representative of the academic registrar's office (responsible for all assessment procedures within the institution). Peer evaluation is usually provided by a colleague/colleagues from other departments who are not directly involved in the course. Nurse educationalists from other institutions and perhaps members of the CNAA, with recognised expertise or interest on aspects of the course, represent the 'experts'. All members of the internal vetting panel receive the course submission document, and each member may be responsible for focusing on specific areas. The CPG includes not only members who have been involved in compiling the submission, but also student

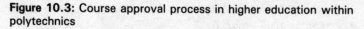

Figure 10.3: Course approval process in higher education within polytechnics

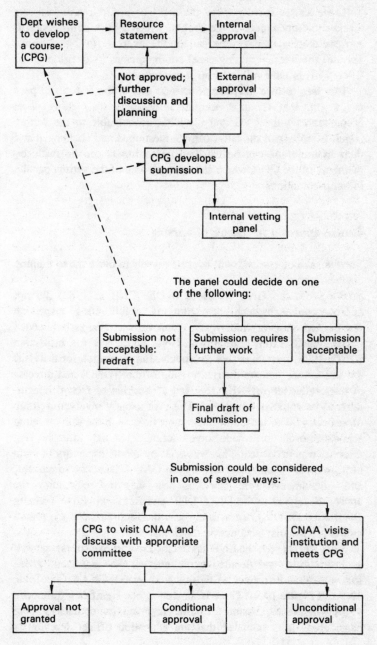

representatives (future consumers) and employers (those who will be receiving the final product).

The exercise usually takes the form of a question-and-answer session, on any aspect of the course, which allows both parties to express their views. At the end of the exercise (a 2- to 4-hour session) the internal vetting panel communicates its decision to the CPG. This is later followed up in writing.

This face-to-face interchange reflects one of the features of peer evaluation, that is, dual accountability, with the vetting panel accountable to the CPG and the CPG accountable to the vetting panel. Members of the latter can be questioned and challenged and their assumptions can be clarified. Also inputs can be made by members of the CPG, which can change some of the vetting panel's initial assumptions.

Course approval in schools of nursing

For the sake of clarity I will confine myself to basic nurse training courses.

Pre-1985, the GNC (replaced by the ENB in 1982) did not approve courses as such but institutions. A full visit of inspection was carried out every four years. Approval was then recommended or continued, rarely withdrawn. GNC guidelines for inspection (GNC, 1976) were available to schools. In preparation for the visit, the institution, i.e. the district nursing officer (DNO) and director of nurse education (DNE), received a checklist of factual information to be completed by them. The visit usually involved a group of inspectors who tended to retain their links with the same training schools in order to provide some continuity. Shortly after the visit a report was produced. This was read by other inspectors (a form of peer review), and discussed by the GNC Education Committee, and amendments were made as necessary before sending the approved version to the DNO, DNE and Regional Nurse Training Committee (RNTC). Very rarely was the report sent to the region unless a particular action was required.

Since April 1985, the ENB has decided to approve courses as well as institutions, and detailed guidelines have been issued. These follow similar principles to those stated by the CNAA (see Table 10.5 and Figure 10.4). There is, however, one significant difference in the way the submission for basic nurse training courses is being considered. It is intended that the education officer (previously

Figure 10.4: ENB course approval process (ENB, 1985)

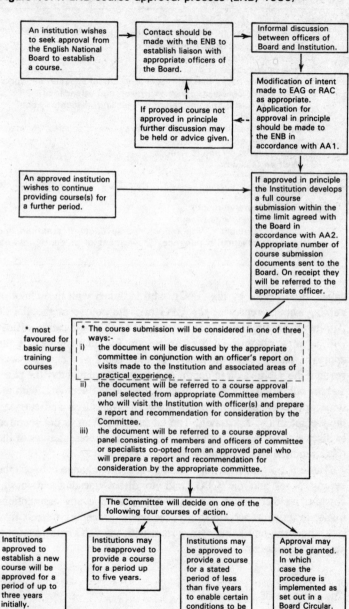

An institution wishes to seek approval from the English National Board to establish a course.

Contact should be made with the ENB to establish liaison with appropriate officers of the Board.

Informal discussion between officers of Board and Institution.

If proposed course not approved in principle further discussion may be held or advice given.

Modification of intent made to EAG or RAC as appropriate. Application for approval in principle should be made to the ENB in accordance with AA1.

An approved institution wishes to continue providing course(s) for a further period.

If approved in principle the Institution develops a full course submission within the time limit agreed with the Board in accordance with AA2. Appropriate number of course submission documents sent to the Board. On receipt they will be referred to the appropriate officer.

* most favoured for basic nurse training courses

* The course submission will be considered in one of three ways:-

i) the document will be discussed by the appropriate committee in conjunction with an officer's report on visits made to the Institution and associated areas of practical experience.

ii) the document will be referred to a course approval panel selected from appropriate Committee members who will visit the Institution with officer(s) and prepare a report and recommendation for consideration by the Committee.

iii) the document will be referred to a course approval panel consisting of members and officers of committee or specialists co-opted from an approved panel who will prepare a report and recommendation for consideration by the appropriate committee.

The Committee will decide on one of the following four courses of action.

Institutions approved to establish a new course will be approved for a period of up to three years initially.

Institutions may be reapproved to provide a course for a period up to five years.

Institutions may be approved to provide a course for a stated period of less than five years to enable certain conditions to be met which will be specified by the Committee.

Approval may not be granted. In which case the procedure is implemented as set out in a Board Circular.

Table 10.5: ENB course approval: information required (ENB, 1985)

A *The training institution*
 1. Name, address, official correspondent, etc.
 2. Educational philosophy/strategy
 3. Educational developments
 4. Relevant courses in the institution
 5. Educational policy-making machinery, communication networks
 6. Educational policies: course admission and attendance
    requirements; student career counselling, discontinuation
    policies, etc.
 7. Staff: staff-student ratios; staff development policies; librarian
    services, etc.
 8. Accommodation and resources
 9. Welfare facilities

B *The course*
 10. Course details
 11. Financial arrangements
 12. Course management team
 13. Course curriculum: integration; course content; structure and
 organisation; practical experience; assessment of students; internal
 evaluation, etc.

called an inspector by the GNC), who is linked with the school of
nursing should represent the CPG and the course at the ENB's
Approvals Committee ((i) in Figure 10.4). The education officer
will write a synopsis of the submission for all members of the
approval panel; three members of that panel are charged with
reading the submission in depth, and on the appointed day the panel
and the education officer will discuss the course document, with the
three appointed panel members answering questions and carrying
the weight of the discussion. The education officer is not required
to discuss the synopsis with the CPG, nor are representatives of the
CPG required to attend the meeting.

There is no provision for a face-to-face interchange between the
vetting panel and the CPG, and no direct question-and-answer
session. Neither group can clarify or challenge any assumptions
made. In terms of accountability, the whole procedure reflects firm
central control and a one-way system with the CPG being accountable to the statutory body.

The purpose of evaluation

According to McCormick and James (1983) the purpose of evaluation is three-fold: evaluation for accountability; evaluation for

professional development and educational improvement; and evaluation for curriculum review. There is an interesting relationship between the first two which also serves to illustrate the political nature of evaluation and brings back into focus the conflicting ideologies of the 'managerial' model of evaluation (represented here by the ENB and the NHS service managers) and the 'professional' model of evaluation (as represented by the CNAA and teachers). Lawton (1984) argues that ideology provides the key to what a group or an institution wants to control as well as to the why and the how. We have already established the connection between evaluation and control. Very simply, knowledge of a system gives power over it. Conflict arises when both 'managers' and 'professionals' claim control.

This brief account of course approval by the CNAA and the ENB seems to indicate that they operate under different ideologies: the CNAA delegates control to professional groups, dispersing accountability and relying on peer evaluation carried out at different levels. The CPG is accountable to the department, depending upon the institution's organisational structure, to the faculty where the department is allocated, and to the general management of the institution, as well as to the validating bodies: CNAA and/or ENB. Within schools of nursing, the ENB exhibits a more direct, centralist and bureaucratic approach with accountability concentrated on a few levels in a hierarchical manner. The DNE is directly accountable for the CPG to the ENB and to a service manager who might be a nurse as in the case of a chief nursing officer or might be an administrator such as in the case of a personnel officer.

It can be argued that the system of validation operating in higher education is more public than that in schools of nursing. This is not surprising. Up till now, schools of nursing have not been asked to give an account. I would argue that this has been a deliberately thought-out strategy. By not asking nurse teachers to give an account of their performance, service managers can keep education under control and in a subservient position. The CNAA is presently involved in devolving responsibility to institutions which demonstrate self-evaluative skills and a degree of professional awareness and development. Devolution has been a slow process, and it has come about partly because of pressure from professional groups which are more accustomed to negotiation and to the development of collegial relationships.

Lawton (1984) expressed concern over the increasing centralism of the DES and suggests that it was the role of professional groups to make such an input into the central authority system. What is certain is that in the journey towards devolution learning has to take place on both sides.

Evaluation, if managed properly, can provide a way for teachers within schools of nursing to gain a foothold in the political arena of decision-making. However. they must give proof of professional maturity by acknowledging that this claim for power and responsibility must be open to inspection: the inspection should be negotiated, democratic and participative.

In the politics of evaluation the issue is represented by who chooses the model of evaluation most suited to the purpose of education. In order for nurse teachers to claim that prerogative, they must demonstrate *responsible professional autonomy* by being more open, and they must prepare themselves thoroughly for the difficult task ahead.

REFERENCES

Becher, A. and Maclure, S. (eds) (1978) *Accountability in education.* NFER, Windsor

Bendall, E.R.D. (1975) *So you passed, nurse.* Royal College of Nursing, London

Carpenter, M. (1978) Managerialism and the division of labour in nursing, in R. Dingwall and J. McIntosh, (eds) *Readings in the sociology of nursing.* Churchill Livingstoke, Edinburgh

Cohen, L. and Manion, L. (1980) *Research methods in education.* Croom Helm, London

Davies, C. (ed.) (1982) *Rewriting nursing history.* Croom Helm, London

Davis, B.D. (ed.) (1983) *Research into nurse education.* Croom Helm, London

Dickinson, S. (1982) The nursing process and the professional status of the nurse. *Nursing Times Occasional Papers.* 78 (16), 61–4

Dodd, A.P. (1973) Towards an understanding of nursing, PhD thesis, University of London

Durrell, L. (1969) in A.G. Thomas (ed.) *Spirit of place.* Faber & Faber, London

Eisner, E.W. (1978) Foreword, in G. Willis (ed.) *Qualitative evaluation: concepts and cases in curriculum criticism.* McCutchan, xi–xvi, Berkeley, CA

English National Board (1985) ENB Approval Process for Courses in Nursing, Midwifery and Health Visiting. 1985/30/MAT

Gallego, A.P. (1983) *Evaluating the school.* Royal College of Nursing, London

General Nursing Council (1976) Checklists for inspectors — hospital approved to participate in training schemes for admission to (A) the Register — General/Sick Children, (B) The Roll — General. (GNC Inspector's private papers)

General Nursing Council (1980) Conditions under which the Council approves schemes of training for the Register and Roll of nurses in England and Wales, 80/11

Kramer, M. (1974) *Reality shock: why nurses leave nursing.* C.V. Mosby, Chicago, Ill.

Lawton, D. (1978) Curriculum evaluation: new approaches, in D. Lawton *et al.* (eds) *Theory and practice of curriculum studies.* Routledge & Kegan Paul, London

Lawton, D. (1984) The tightening grip: growth of central control of the school curriculum. Bedford Way Papers. University of London, Institute of Education

McCormick, R. and James, M. (1983) *Curriculum evaluation in schools.* Croom Helm, London

Macdonald, B. (1974) Evaluation and the control of education, in *Innovation, evaluation, research and the problem of control* (Safari project). CARE, University of East Anglia, Norwich

Musgrove, F. (1973) Research on the sociology of the school and of teaching, in W. Taylor, (ed.) *Research perspectives in education.* Routledge & Kegan Paul, London

Parlett, M. and Hamilton, D. (1972) Evaluation as illumination: a new approach to the study of innovatory programmes. Occasional Paper 9. Centre for Research in the Educational Sciences, University of Edinburgh. Reprinted in D. Hamilton *et al.* (eds) (1977) *Beyond the numbers game.* Macmillan, London

Pring, R. (1984) The problems of confidentiality, in M. Skilbeck (ed.) *Evaluating the curriculum in the eighties.* Hodder & Stoughton, London

Rapoport, R.N. (1970) Three dilemmas in action research. *Human Relations, 23,* 499–513

Report of the Committee on Nursing (1972) Chairman: Prof. A Briggs. HMSO Cmnd 5115

Report of the Committee on Senior Nursing Staff (1966) Chairman: B. Salmon, HMSO, London

Schon, D. (1971) *Beyond the stable state: public and private learning in a changing society.* Temple Smith, London, p. 51

Simons, H. (1977) Building a social contract, in N. Norris (ed.) *Safari: theory in practice papers, two.* CARE, University of East Anglia, Norwich

Simons, H. (1980a) Process evaluation in schools, in C. Lacey and D. Lawton (eds) *Accountability in evaluation.* Methuen, London

Simons, H. (1980b) The evaluative school. *Forum, 22* (2) 55–7

Walker, R. (1977) Descriptive methodology, in N. Norris (ed.) *Safari: theory in practice papers, two.* CARE, University of East Anglia, Norwich

BIBLIOGRAPHY

CNAA (1979) *Developments in partnership in validation.* CNAA, London

CNAA (1982) *Principles and regulations for the award of the Council's first degrees and Diploma of Higher Education.* CNAA, London

11

Classroom Instruction and Clinical Opportunity in Student Nurse Training: Integration and Measurement

D.C. Lewin and K. Jacka

INTRODUCTION

The main aim of the Clinical Learning Project at the Nursing Education Research Unit, King's College (Chelsea), is to describe and illuminate the clinical (ward-based) learning of student nurses. Learning depends upon *experience*, which itself depends upon *opportunity*: here we use 'opportunity' to refer to the amount and variety of clinical material present in the group of training wards to which the student is allocated as she progresses through the stages of her training. Clinical opportunity is therefore the necessary precursor and basis of clinical learning.

However, theoretical knowledge is equally requisite: without theoretical instruction, in the classroom, on the ward, or in both environments, the student will learn little from her clinical encounters. Then again, the instruction may be good in itself and yet bear little fruit; it depends on several factors, and experienced nurse educators are agreed that an important one is the degree of integration between classroom and ward, i.e. the degree to which a given item of theoretical instruction is linked with corresponding clinical material encountered by the student in her placements.

There were three elements in the terms of reference of the project, three questions to consider: to ascertain what student nurses learn in clinical learning areas, what they should learn, and what factors promote or inhibit clinical learning. Any serious attempt to answer these questions would require an investigation of both classroom and ward, and the experiences of students within them; likewise any discussion of experience would most naturally, as we indicated before, first attend to the structure — the possibilities of experience — before turning to the actualities of individual learning careers. The researchers addressed themselves to all three questions, and reported upon them, but this chapter is concerned only with the first question (what students learn in clinical learning areas) and with clinical opportunity rather than clinical experience.

In the exploratory phase of the project, undertaken in eleven schools of nursing, it was found that clinical learning problems were similar, regardless of hospital type, training scheme or geographical location; i.e. there was a core of problems common to all programmes, and the quality of training students received depended very much on how well or how badly they were handled (Leach and Lewin, 1981). Given a common core of problems, it follows that there is little to be gained from carrying out an extensive and therefore necessarily superficial study; better to concentrate on a few hospitals and investigate in depth within them the opportunities and actualities of clinical experience. In the second phase, therefore, the research team chose three cohorts ('sets') of student nurses, one from each of three schools of nursing, and followed each trainee (72 in all) from the beginning of training until qualification. There were other elements in the research design, but the cohort study was the centrepiece. The reasoning behind this research design derived from the fact that clinical learning occurs within the life of an individual student: each student has a unique learning career, and it can be difficult, even misleading, to make deductions about the learning of an individual over a short interval of time within the three years of training.

BACKGROUND AND METHODS

The schools were located in a district general hospital in a London suburb (modified modular scheme): Hospital 1; a London teaching hospital (modular scheme): Hospital 2; and a district general hospital in the provinces (block scheme): Hospital 3. The study commenced with 87 students, there was some attrition (average: 17%) and 72 completed the course. At Hospital 1, 22 student nurses completed the course; at Hospital 2, 30; and at Hospital 3, 20.

Primary data

The main sources of primary data were as follows.

(a) Tutorial staff

Each school of nursing sent the research team a copy of the relevant timetable at the end of every block or module. The whole set was ultimately collated and then analysed, and the contents were finally classified into 27 categories. The purpose of classification was to illuminate and to facilitate comparison, using familiar terminology to devise categories that were neither too coarse nor too detailed, and which were both exhaustive and mutually exclusive. With a structure as complex and as dependent on personal judgement and idiosyncrasy as a training programme, there are sure to be problems of classification; for the most part, however, they were minor, enabling the final classification to be quite good enough for making useful comparisons.

(b) Allocation officers

Throughout the study, the three nursing allocation officers provided the researchers with detailed information about the allocation of student nurses in training.

(c) Ward sisters

Ward and departmental sisters of all training areas were interviewed, and informed the research team on a variety of matters including the clinical emphases of their wards.

(d) Observation

Wards were visited (often more than once) by the research team: during these visits, the researchers looked at many aspects of the ward and studied the nursing notes ('Kardex'), attending especially to the patient diagnoses.

Classroom instruction

Here we consider the analysis of theoretical instruction. Table 11.1 shows an example of how classroom material in a two-week study block was analysed. This mode of analysis was employed for all study blocks and modules in each of the training schemes.

We next isolate the clinical component of instruction, first because it is of interest in itself, and secondly because it is only this clinical component that we shall use when we come to consider the integration of classroom and ward. By 'clinical component' we mean instruction specific to the nursing of particular kinds of

Table 11.1: Analysis of classroom material in a two-week study block (Hospital 1, Block 1)

Topic	Hours	%
Alimentary nursing	11	19
Cardiovascular/circulatory nursing	9	16
Study	9	16
Tests and assessments	6	10
Introduction to nursing research	5	9
Endocrine nursing	5	9
Respiratory nursing	4	7
Neurological nursing	4	7
Fire prevention	2	3
Genito-urinary nursing	1	2
Management exercise	1	2
Project work	1	2
Total	58	102[a]

[a]Percentages rounded to nearest whole number

patients. In Table 11.1, for example, it includes alimentary, cardiovascular, endocrine, respiratory, neurological and genito-urinary nursing, but excludes study periods, tests and assessments, an introduction to nursing research, fire prevention, management exercise and project work. In our study, the average clinical component of classroom instruction in three schools of nursing was 73%.

CATEGORIES OF CLINICAL DIAGNOSES

Numbers of training wards

In Hospital 1 training was concentrated on relatively few wards (13); in Hospital 2 there was a large number (37); in Hospital 3 the number was intermediate (22). There were thus 72 training wards in all. Two (in Hospital 2) were not visited by the research team (for logistic reasons). One of these specialised in endocrine, metabolic and genetic problems; the other was a busy, high-dependency intensive-therapy and coronary-care unit. For these two only, clinical data derived solely from information provided by the ward sisters. There was a close second accord between the sisters' description of ward specialties and the estimates of the researchers as a result of their own observation.

Patients

To estimate the clinical opportunities available to students, the researchers collected diagnostic information on a large number of patients in the training wards. For the following reasons, we believe this gives a picture of student clinical opportunity which is sufficiently accurate for our purposes.

(a) Probability sampling

The total of patients observed on any given ward was approximately proportional to the number of students allocated to that ward over the three-year period. For example, if on one ward, Andover, the number of patients observed was 74, and on Axminster it was 25, this reflects the fact that about three times as many students passed through the former as the latter. (To put it another way: a student was three times as likely to be assigned to Andover as to Axminster.) The most used wards were therefore also the most accurately estimated. (Note: ward names are fictitious.)

(b) Stability

The visits were usually made near the middle of the placement. If a placement were for ten weeks and the average patient stay was only one week, then clearly we have only a small sample of the student's experience. However, this was of little importance, since observation confirmed the sisters' claims that the clinical picture of a ward would remain fairly steady over time.

(c) Nursing notes ('Kardex')

Although several authors (Selmanoff and Walker, 1964; Healy and McGurk, 1966; Georgopoulos and Jackson, 1970; Lelean, 1973) have criticised the quality of ward communication and recording, mentioning especially the daily nursing report, the researchers found the nursing notes to be reasonably clear and reliable as a *diagnostic* record. They were used as the main comprehensive source of diagnostic data. (On each ward the researchers independently checked a sample of diagnoses.)

Each patient was given a diagnostic category derived from the International Statistical Classification of Diseases. Up to two categories were used for each patient, if required. Seventeen categories were used, but these were reduced, by conflation, to a final set of 5, as shown in Table 11.2. 'Social problems' was used only for patients whose admission was purely for social reasons.

Table 11.2: Diagnosis categories

Original classification	Final classification
Diseases of lower alimentary tract; diseases of higher alimentary tract	Alimentary nursing
Cardiac disorders; circulatory disorders; lymphatic disorders	Cardiovascular and circulatory nursing
Breast disorders; disorders of female reproductive organs	Gynaecological nursing
Conditions of renal system; conditions of male reproductive organs	Genito-urinary nursing
Conditions of skeletal system; dental extractions	Orthopaedic nursing
Conditions of the skin; plastic surgery, burns	Dermatological nursing

'Other conditions' was used for diagnoses that defied classification. These numbered 47 out of 4010 (1.2%) and included patients admitted for terminal care, collapse (query cause) metastatic tumours of unknown primary, pyrexias of unknown origin, carcinomatosis, a child with persistent screaming, and a small number of infective and genetic conditions (e.g. haemolytic streptococcal infection and Down's syndrome).

Analysis was based on medical diagnoses. Many nurses would like to move away from this kind of emphasis, but the research team decided to hold to the way in which patients were actually categorised on the training wards since otherwise comparisons would have been extremely difficult. Table 11.3 shows aggregates for all patients observed and all diagnostic categories.

Table 11.3: Summary of diagnostic data

Hospital	Visits	Wards	Patients	Diagnostic categories
1	34	13	726	1078
2	44	35	823	1257
3	48	22	995	1675
Total	126	70	2544	4010

Roper (1976) noted that 39% of patients in a general hospital had more than one medical diagnostic label. Our figure is comparable, although somewhat higher (58%).

241

NUMERICAL ANALYSIS OF CLINICAL DATA

Diagnoses, by ward

Numbers and percentages for each category were calculated for all training wards. Below we discuss one of the wards; the figures are presented in Table 11.4.

Table 11.4: Diagnosis, by ward (Hospital number: 1; ward name: Aberdeen; label: female surgical; beds: 27; visits: 1)

Diagnosis	Number	%
Gynaecology/breast disorders	26	81.3
Alimentary	2	6.3
Cardiovascular/circulatory	1	3.1
Endocrine	1	3.1
Dermatology/plastic surgery/burns	1	3.1
Social admissions	1	3.1
Genito-urinary	0	0.0
Neuromedicine/neurosurgery	0	0.0
Orthopaedics/dental	0	0.0
Eyes/ear, nose and throat	0	0.0
Psychiatry	0	0.0
Respiratory	0	0.0
Other conditions	0	0.0
Total	32	100.0

Hospital 1: Aberdeen — a female surgical gynaecology ward. The figures show that 81.3% of diagnostic categories pertained to gynaecology/breast disorders, with small proportions relating to the alimentary tract, the skin, cardiovascular/circulatory and endocrine systems, and social problems.

Although most patients were diagnosed as having gynaecological problems (infertility, menorrhagia, fibroids, carcinoma of the cervix, an ectopic pregnancy, and prolapses of various kinds), one had a burst abdomen following surgery to the large bowel, another an appendectomy, a third diabetes, a fourth anaemia, a fifth was troubled by a skin rash, and an exhausted pregnant young woman, with a known gynaecological history, was admitted on account of her social problems.

Diagnoses, by hospital

Table 11.5 displays aggregated data. The key figures are the percentages in each row; as already explained, these figures incorporate the fact that some wards are used more than others. The table takes no account of individual student variation: it gives, in effect, a picture of the relative proportions of clinical conditions that *on average* a student could expect to encounter throughout her training.

INTEGRATION OF CLASSROOM AND WARD

In this section we shall be examining the integration of learning opportunity between classroom and ward, an aspect of training that is intrinsically more complex and difficult to disentangle. In this case one cannot commence with aggregates — they tell one nothing: it is individual sequence that is all important. Even with a small number of training wards (as in Hospital 1) a sequence such as: Block 1, Aysgarth Ward; Block 2, Andover Ward, Axminster Ward; Block 3, Aberdeen Ward, could be quite different in respect of integration from: Block 1, Axminster Ward; Block 2, Aberdeen Ward, Aysgarth Ward; Block 3, Andover Ward. Here the only path to insight is by examining the training sequence for each student and by estimating in some reasonable way the amount of integration opportunity that the training scheme has achieved. In this section we do just this; the ultimate results of analysis turn out to be surprisingly clear and definite.

All members of a cohort came together for class instruction, but only a small number (typically between one and four) were allocated to the same training ward. The data therefore contained three sequences of theoretical instruction (one for each school) and 72 sequences (22, 30, 20) of clinical allocation. These data were examined in the light of the assumptions informing the modular system of training. Indices of integration between theory and practice were computed for individual trainees, and these were aggregated to produce indices for hospitals. The results were used to answer the following fundamental questions in nursing training:

(a) Within each hospital, what is the degree of equality of educational opportunity (in respect of integration)?
(b) For each hospital, what is the maximum level of integration which the organisation of training makes possible?

243

Table 11.5: Diagnosis, by hospital

Hospital	Alimentary		Cardiovascular/Circulatory		Gynaecology/Breast disorders		Endocrine		Psychiatry		Respiratory		Genito-urinary		Neuromedicine/Neurosurgery		Social admissions		Orthopaedic/Dental		Eyes/ENT		Dermatology/Plastic surgery/Burns		Other		Total	
	No.	%	No.	%	No.	%	No.	%	No.	%	No.	%	No.	%	No.	%	No.	%	No.	%	No.	%	No.	%	No.	%	No.	%
H1	207	19.2	207	19.2	41	3.8	46	4.3	32	3.0	97	9.0	110	10.2	140	13.0	18	1.7	113	10.5	19	1.8	36	3.3	12	1.1	1078	100.1
H2	168	13.4	144	11.4	126	10.0	49	3.9	40	3.2	113	9.0	91	7.2	165	13.1	20	1.6	196	15.6	69	5.5	59	4.7	17	1.4	1257	100.0
H3	251	15.0	310	18.5	69	4.1	83	5.0	36	2.1	162	9.7	128	8.2	179	10.7	7	0.4	314	18.7	46	2.7	62	3.7	18	1.1	1675	99.9
Total	626	15.6	661	16.5	236	5.9	178	4.4	108	2.7	372	9.3	339	8.5	484	12.1	45	1.1	623	15.5	134	3.3	157	3.9	47	1.2	4010	100.0

(c) Aggregating the trainee data for each cohort, what is the *actual* level of integration reached within each hospital?

(d) Hospital 1 describes its training scheme as 'modified modular'; Hospital 2 describes its training scheme as 'modular'; Hospital 3 describes its training scheme as 'block'. In the light of the answers to (a), (b) and (c), are these self-descriptions accurate?

Student profiles

There were clear indications of stability (low standard deviation) within each hospital. It was therefore decided to use a 50% random sample. This consisted of: 13 student nurses from Hospital 1, 17 student nurses from Hospital 2, and 10 student nurses from Hospital 3. For each of these trainees a profile or flow chart was compiled. The vertical axis exhibits the sequence of theory and practice as encountered by the student (holidays were also included). The horizontal axis itemises a composite list of diagnostic categories; these were chosen as constituting the most accurate and succinct set for describing jointly the clinical elements occurring in both classroom and ward.

Table 11.6 gives an example of one of these profiles. A few notes of explanation will help in giving detail and in elucidating certain recondite aspects of the presentations.

(1) The list on the horizontal axis derives from the syllabus analysis described above ('Classroom instruction'), supplemented by the ward analysis of clinical conditions. It is essentially a list of nursing and diagnostic categories covering all three classroom curricula, with some additions and rephrasing to accommodate the kinds of diagnostic classification encountered on the wards. Not all of the categories occurred in every hospital. For example, Hospitals 2 and 3 included aspects of radiotherapy nursing, which were not present in Hospital 1. Another example is 'social admissions', a category deriving from the ward analysis; this category did relate to some elements of classroom instruction, but was not itemised in these terms. Note, however, that these more irregular categories (radiotherapy nursing, social admissions) were all of small magnitude and therefore would not have much effect on any aggregate measure of integration, however classified and scored, and the larger categories were effectively unequivocal in classification and uniform in occurrence.

245

Table 11.6: Student-nurse profile, Hospital 1, Nurse 101

	Accident & emergency	Infectious diseases	Psychiatry	Social admissions	Dermatology/Plastic surgery/Burns	Eyes/Ear, nose & throat	Alimentary	Cardiovascular/Circulatory	Gynaecology/Breast disorders	Endocrine	Respiratory	Genito-urinary	Paediatrics	Neurology	Orthopaedics/Dental	Care of the elderly	Theatre/Anaesthetics	ITU	Total (%)
Block 1			3			2	19	16		9	7	2		7	2				60
Andover			2	6	7	1	10	22		8	18	6		15	6				99
Abingdon					8		34	11		2	6	28		2					100
Block 2							36	26	4	4	11								81
Annual leave																			
4 weeks																			
Block 3						5				17	8			29		14	8		73
Ascot			16		3	3	3	57	5	6	3	5		13	6				101
Axminster			3	3	2	6	3	6		3	5	3		56	5				99
Adlestrop						2	47	12		3		7		5					99
Theatres																			
Annual leave																			
4 weeks																			
Block 4			2							32				26		2	↔3	8	73

Block 5	6				18				85
Psychiatry	10 ↔								
Obstetrics									
Aysgarth	6	25	36	8	35	26			99
Block 6	2	2	9	18	2	21	9	27	64
Annual leave 4 weeks									
Block 7	2	16	6	23	5	21			87
Aberdeen	3	3	1	34	6	3	3	4	5	99
Ambleside	2	2	1	15	81	4	25	5	12	102
Accident & emergency						4	4		12
Amersham	4		2	11		2	7		101
Arundel	5	4	2	20	18	9	18	32	2	99
Block 8	3	8	8	3		2	9	5	13	58
Annual leave 4 weeks									
Block 9	1		2	13	9	4		11		30
Aldeburgh	1	1	31	20		7	6	10	12	100
Annual leave 2 weeks									
Balancing modules 1–5									
Ashington	6	3	1	9	16	8	23	3	23	5	98

(2) The figures in the cells are percentages (nearest whole number). For Table 11.6 only (Hospital 1, Nurse 101) we have written in the row totals. For Block 1 this is 60%. This means that the *clinical* elements of instruction in this block accounted for 60% of the total time (19% alimentary, 16% cardiovascular, etc.). The corresponding figure for Block 2 is 81%. The reader will recall that the average for all blocks/modules for all hospitals is 73%.

For the wards the figures in each row refer to the proportions of diagnostic categories of patients that one would expect to encounter. For Andover Ward these proportions were 3% psychiatry, 6% social admissions, etc. The total here is, of course, always 100% or thereabouts.

(3) The specialist placements of psychiatry and obstetrics were excluded from this analysis for two reasons:

(a) the research team considerd it inappropriate to observe in some sensitive areas associated with these specialties;

(b) it was known that in all three hospitals a study day system operated, enabling theory and practice to be closely integrated. By ignoring these areas we are subtracting a constant element, and therefore the realisation of our ultimate aim — a comparison of differences — will not be affected.

(4) Although we have excluded psychiatry and obstetrics placements, as being self-contained units of high integration, we have taken note of the occasional situation where one of these specialist placements is anticipated by the school, either by accident or design, and, in effect, some orientation lectures are given; a double arrow symbolises the integration.

Scoring for contiguity

The core of the argument for the modular system of nurse training was that a student was most likely to benefit if classroom instruction in a given area (say cardiology) was supported by clinical material on the ward occurring fairly near in time (either before or after). Although plausible, and in accord with the judgement of experienced teachers, we are not here concerned with the truth of this contention, but only with the facts. What happened: to what extent did such a linking of theory and practice occur in the training sequences of the students under investigation?

To get an idea of this we devised the simplest kind of scoring

Table 11.7: Contiguity scoring: example 1

Nurse 101	Alimentary	Score	Paediatrics	Score
Block 1	19 ⌐			
Andover	10 ⌐→ 1			
Abingdon	34 ⌐			
Block 2	36 ⌐→ 1			
Annual leave 4 weeks				
Block 3				
Ascot	3			
Axminister				
Adlestrop	47		5	
Theatres				
Annual leave 4 weeks				
Block 4				
Block 5			26	
Psychiatry				
Obstetrics				
Aysgarth	36		0 ↕ ⌐	
Block 6			8 ⌐→ 1	
Annual leave 4 weeks				
Block 7				
Aberdeen	6			
Ambleside	34			
Accident & emergency				
Amersham	2			
Arundel	2			
Block 8				
Annual leave 4 weeks				
Block 9	2 ⌐			
Aldeburgh	31 ⌐→ 1			
Annual leave 2 weeks				
Balancing modules 1–5				
Ashington	9			
Total score		3		1

system, in which a point was awarded each time an element of classroom instruction was immediately preceded or followed by an essentially similar element of clinical opportunity. The system is most easily understood by a few examples.

In Table 11.7 we have set down a part of the information relating to Nurse 101.

(1) In the column headed 'Alimentary' we see that 19% of classroom instruction in Block 1 relates to this topic. The nurse is then allocated to Andover Ward which has 10% of clinical material relating to alimentary nursing. This pair of adjacent figures (19, 10) therefore generates a score of 1. Similarly, for Block 2 (36%), which is preceded by an allocation to Abingdon

249

Table 11.8: Contiguity scoring: example 2

Nurse 201	Alimentary	Score
Module 1	11	
Bideford	5	1
Annual leave (1 week)		
Module 2	15	1
Bodmin	3	1
Module 3		
Banbury	9	1
Module 4	13	
Burwell	64	1
Annual leave (2 weeks)		1
Module 5	5	
Bridlington	14	1
Module 6		
Psychiatry		
Module 7		
Obstetrics		
Annual leave (1 week)		
Module 8	5	
Biggleswade	20	1
Annual leave (2 weeks)		1
Module 9	16	
Balmoral	34	1
Module 10	11	1
Blackburn		
Senior nursing module	4	
Theatre		
Braintree		
Barking	24	
Management module 1		
Annual leave (2 weeks)		
Bromley	11	
Managment module 2	5	1
Total score		12

ward containing 34% of alimentary clinical material, this sequence also generates a score of 1; and near the bottom of the page we have a further sequence (Block 9, Aldeburgh), generating a final score of 1. Altogether, there is a total score of 3 units for this diagnostic category.

Occasionally there is a doubtful case. One could argue, for instance, that the sequence Block 2 (36%), annual leave (4 weeks), Block 3 (0%), Ascot (3%) justifies a score of 1 unit, in that there is no *allocation* intervening between Block 2 and Ascot. If the sequence had been Block 2 (36%), Block 3 (0%), Ascot (3%), we would have scored it, but in the above situation we judged that the actual sequence was too attenuated in regard to integration to justify a score.

(2) In the column headed 'Paediatrics', the double arrow is present because Aysgarth is a paediatric ward. Being adjacent to Block 6 (8%) this generates a score of 1.

(3) Table 11.8 presents one column of information ('Alimentary') for Nurse 201, and one can see how the modular sequence of theory and practice makes possible a much larger score (12) than was achieved by Nurse 101. Note that in scoring for Nurse 201 we often span a period of annual leave, but in all cases the period of leave was short and would not, we judged, lead to any substantial break in continuity.

Contiguity scoring: results

Aspects of variation

Tables 11.9–11 summarise the contiguity scores for all 40 of the trainees investigated, and enable us to examine, in respect of integration between theory and practice, the variation in experience within the group of students. Within any one hospital there are two possible kinds of variation: that in the total scores of individual students; and that in scores for each of the diagnostic categories.

(a) Comparison of aggregates. There are two ways (each of them useful) of quantifying variation within a group: the ratio of maximum to minimum; and the ratio of standard deviation to arithmetic mean (coefficient of variation). We shall discuss each in turn.

(i) In Hospital 1 the highest aggregate score is 34 (Nurse 115); the lower is 25 (Nurse 123). In Hospital 2 the highest aggregate score is 82 (Nurse 231); the lowest is 58 (Nurse 227). In Hospital 3 the highest aggregate score is 43 (Nurse 301); the lowest is 27 (Nurse 317). Table 11.12 shows that the most favourable allocation sequence in Hospital 1 generates 36% more contiguity points than the least favourable. Using this index, Hospital 2 is slightly behind Hospital 1, with Hospital 3 showing a substantially greater degree of inequality.

(ii) In Hospital 1 the mean aggregate score is 29.2 and the variation is 2.38 (as measured by the standard deviation). In Hospital 2 the mean aggregate score is 69.9 and the standard deviation is 7.40. In Hospital 3 the mean aggregate score is 33.1 and the

251

Table 11.9: Hospital 1: contiguity scores

Nurse	Accident & emergency	Psychiatry	Dermatology/Plastic surgery/Burns	Eyes/Ear, nose & throat	Alimentary	Cardiovascular/Circulatory	Gynaecology/Breast disorders	Endocrine	Respiratory	Genito-urinary	Paediatrics	Neuromedicine/Neurosurgery	Orthopaedics/Dental	Care of the elderly	Theatre/Anaesthetics	Total: contiguous relationships
101	0	1	0	2	3	4	1	4	2	2	1	4	1	0	1	26
103	0	1	1	2	3	4	2	4	2	2	1	4	1	0	1	28
105	0	0	1	3	3	4	0	4	2	2	1	5	2	0	1	28
107	0	2	1	3	3	4	1	3	2	2	0	5	2	0	1	29
109	0	1	1	2	3	4	1	5	2	2	1	6	1	1	0	29
111	0	0	1	2	3	4	1	5	2	2	1	6	0	1	0	28
113	0	2	1	2	3	4	0	4	2	2	1	7	2	1	0	31
115	1	2	1	2	3	4	4	4	3	2	0	6	2	1	0	34
117	0	1	1	1	3	4	1	5	2	2	1	6	1	1	0	30
119	1	2	1	2	3	3	1	4	2	2	1	5	2	0	1	30
121	1	2	1	2	3	4	4	3	2	2	0	5	2	0	1	32
123	0	1	1	0	3	4	3	3	2	2	0	4	1	0	1	25
125	1	0	1	2	3	4	1	3	2	2	1	6	2	0	1	29
x̄	0.31	1.15	0.92	1.92	3.00	3.92	1.54	3.92	2.10	2.00	0.69	5.31	1.46	0.38	0.62	29.23
s	0.48	0.80	0.27	0.76	0.0	0.28	1.33	0.76	0.28	0.0	0.48	0.95	0.66	0.51	0.51	2.38

Table 11.10: Hospital 2: contiguity scores

Nurse	Trauma	Psychiatry	Dermatology/Plastic surgery/Burns	Eyes/Ear, nose & throat	Alimentary	Cardiovascular/Circulatory	Gynaecology/Breast disorders	Endocrine	Respiratory	Genito-urinary	Neuromedicine/Neurosurgery	Orthopaedics/Dental	Total: contiguous relationships
201	1	4	5	5	12	12	1	4	6	11	8	7	76
203	1	3	7	7	12	12	2	5	7	9	8	7	80
205	1	3	6	5	10	11	1	3	5	6	5	3	59
207	1	4	7	4	10	13	2	6	6	10	6	4	73
209	1	3	2	4	12	12	1	4	6	11	5	5	66
211	1	2	6	6	12	10	2	1	4	8	3	4	59
213	1	5	5	9	13	11	1	4	5	9	6	5	75
215	1	3	8	5	12	12	0	4	7	11	7	7	78
217	1	5	5	3	13	12	1	3	6	9	6	7	70
219	1	3	7	5	8	12	2	6	5	11	6	5	72
221	1	3	3	3	10	14	3	4	5	13	4	4	62
223	1	4	3	3	11	10	0	5	6	9	6	5	74
225	1	2	6	6	12	15	2	4	5	9	7	6	69
227	1	3	4	2	8	12	2	3	7	10	3	4	58
229	1	3	4	2	12	14	1	3	5	10	7	5	68
231	1	3	5	5	14	14	2	6	7	12	7	7	82
233	1	2	5	1	10	12	3	5	5	11	7	5	67
$\bar{x}$	1	3.23	5.23	4.4	11.23	12.2	1.52	4.11	5.70	9.94	5.94	5.29	69.9
s	0	0.90	1.56	2.0	1.67	1.39	0.87	1.31	0.91	1.63	1.51	1.31	7.40

Table 11.11: Hospital 3: contiguity scores

Nurse	Pre- and post-operative care	Radiotherapy	Psychiatry	Dermatology/Plastic surgery/Burns	Eyes/Ear, nose & throat	Alimentary	Cardiovascular/Circulatory	Gynaecology/Breast disorders	Endocrine	Respiratory	Genito-urinary	Paediatrics	Neuromedicine/Neurosurgery	Orthopaedics/Dental	Care of the elderly	Total: contiguous relationships
301	4	1	0	0	2	7	8	1	4	4	2	2	3	4	1	43
303	5	1	1	2	2	4	8	1	3	3	1	1	3	3	0	38
305	3	0	2	1	1	4	6	3	2	1	2	0	0	2	1	28
307	4	0	2	1	0	5	7	2	3	3	2	1	2	3	0	35
309	2	0	2	1	1	4	6	2	2	2	1	0	2	3	0	29
311	2	0	1	1	2	4	6	2	3	3	2	0	2	2	1	30
313	2	0	2	1	1	4	5	2	1	2	4	2	3	3	1	31
315	2	0	2	1	1	5	8	0	3	4	2	1	4	2	1	38
317	2	0	2	1	1	4	6	1	2	2	2	0	2	2	1	27
319	4	0	1	0	1	4	7	1	1	3	0	1	2	3	0	32
x̄	3.0	0.2	1.5	1.0	1.2	4.5	6.7	1.5	2.4	2.7	2.0	0.8	2.3	2.7	0.6	33.1
s	1.15	0.42	0.71	0.67	0.63	0.97	1.06	0.85	0.97	0.95	0.82	0.79	1.06	0.67	0.52	5.22

Table 11.12: Aggregate scores: extremes

Hospital	Maximum aggregate	Minimum aggregate	Ratio max ÷ min
1	34	25	1.36
2	82	58	1.41
3	43	27	1.59

Table 11.13: Aggregate scores: comparison of means

Hospital	Mean	Standard deviation	Ratio (standard deviation ÷ mean)
1	29.2	2.38	0.08
2	69.9	7.40	0.11
3	33.1	5.22	0.16

standard deviation is 5.22. The order of precedence is as before; each of the two methods of quantification tells much the same story: only in Hospital 3 is there substantial variation (inequality), and even there it is not very large.

(b) Comparison without each category. Unfavourable unequality (for an individual) occurs when there is a systematic trend of low integration scores across a large number of categories. This will give a low aggregate score (e.g. Nurse 317). However, one can have variation without inequality of aggregates. As an example, consider the following (extracted from Table 11.9).

	Alimentary	Endocrine	Sub-total
Nurse 207	10	6	16
Nurse 209	12	4	16

The sub-totals are the same, even though there is variation.

(i) A glance at Tables 11.9–11 indicates that the variation (best measured by the ratio $s/\bar{x}$) tends to be small for the high-scoring categories such as 'Alimentary' and 'Cardiovascular', and comparatively large for the low-scoring categories such as 'Psychiatry'.

(ii) An *overall* index of this kind of variation is best achieved by

Table 11.14: Variation within a category

Hospital	Mean of $\bar{x}$ values	Mean of s values	Index of overall variation [(ii) ÷ (i)]
1	1.95	0.54	0.28
2	5.82	1.26	0.22
3	2.21	0.82	0.37

computing a ratio of *average* standard deviation to *average* mean.

These data are summarised in Table 11.14. Hospital 2 has the least variation (the greatest degree of *sameness* of experience), Hospital 3 the most variation, and Hospital 1 lies in between.

(c) Comparison between hospitals. The previous section considered aspects of *variation*. Here we wish to compare hospitals in regard to the *magnitude* of integration scores. The information is summarised in Table 11.15.

(i) The analysis required 17 distinct categories in all. Hospital 1 required 15 categories; Hospital 2, 12; and Hospital 3, 15.
(ii) The figures in the body of the table are abstracted from Tables 11.9–12. They are average integration scores per student for a given category.
(iii) The pattern is clear:
  (a) For almost all categories the H2 score is much larger than either of the other two.
  (b) Scores for H1 and H3 are often similar in size.
(iv) Table 11.16 gives the mean scores. The three figures (29.2, 69.9, 33.1) may be taken as indices of integration (contiguity) for the three different hospitals.
(v) Alternatively the figures can be transformed into ratios (Table 11.17).

Estimate of uptake

The previous scoring system used only the notion of contiguity of theory and practice, and this minimal assumption is sufficient for a basic comparison of educational opportunity. For a more plausible estimate of likely *uptake* of educational possibilities, however (a combination of opportunity itself plus facilitation), the notion of

Table 11.15: Inter-hospital comparisons (mean scores)

Hospital	Accident & emergency/Trauma	Psychiatry	Dermatology/Plastic surgery/Burns	Eyes/Ear, nose & throat	Alimentary	Cardiovascular/Circulatory	Gynaecology/Breast disorders	Endocrine	Respiratory	Genito-urinary	Paediatrics	Neuromedicine/Neurosurgery	Orthopaedics/Dental	Care of the elderly	Theatre/Anaesthetics	Pre- and post-operative care	Radiotherapy	Totals
H1	0.31	1.15	0.92	1.92	3.00	3.92	1.54	3.92	2.10	2.00	0.69	5.31	1.46	0.38	0.62	—	—	29.2
H2	1.00	3.23	5.23	4.40	11.23	12.20	1.52	4.11	5.70	9.94	—	5.94	5.29	—	—	—	—	69.9
H3	—	1.50	1.00	1.20	4.50	6.70	1.50	2.40	2.70	2.00	0.80	2.30	2.70	0.60	—	3.00	0.20	33.1

Table 11.16: Mean scores

Hospital	Total score
1	29.2
2	69.9
3	33.1

Table 11.17: Ratios

Comparison	Ratio
H1/H3	0.88
H2/H1	2.39
H2/H3	2.11

proportion should be included. It seems wrong to score identically the following two (hypothetical) situations (for the category of cardiovascular nursing):

(a) Nurse A has 1% of lecture time and 50% of clinical opportunity.
(b) Nurse B has 40% of lecture time and 50% of clinical opportunity.

In order to derive a more plausible estimate of the likely uptake of educational possibilities, the links between theoretical instruction and clinical opportunity were reanalysed. A 'good match' was where there was not only contiguity, but also a good relationship of proportion. Specifically, the ratio of theory to clinical experience had to lie between 0.5 and 2.0 for a score of 2. Below 0.5, or above 2.0, the score was 1. Examples of this more complex scoring are given in Table 11.18.

For Nurse 101 ('Alimentary') the link Block 1-Andover has a ratio of 19/10 (= 1.9). This is greater than 0.5 and less than 2.0 and therefore generates a score of 2, whereas the link Block 9-Aldeburgh has a ratio of 2/31 (= 0.06). This is less than 0.5 and therefore generates a score of 1.

Where relationships were known to exist between theory and practice, but where the extent of the practice was unspecified (designated by connecting arrows in the student profiles; for example with Nurse 101 in respect of operating theatre and psychiatry experiences), the notion of contiguity alone was acknowledged and a score of 1 was awarded.

Table 11.18: Complex scoring: example

Nurse 101	Alimentary	Score	Nurse 201	Alimentary	Score
Block 1	19 } → 2		Module 1	11 } → 1	
Andover	10		Bideford	5	
Abingdon	34 } → 2		Annual leave	} → 1	
Block 2	36		(1 week)		
Annual leave			Module 2	15 } → 1	
(4 weeks)			Bodmin	3	
Block 3			Module 3		
Ascot	3		Banbury	9 } → 2	
Axminster			Module 4	13	
Aldestrop	47		Burwell	64 } → 1	
Theatres			Annual leave	} → 1	
Annual leave			(2 weeks)		
(4 weeks)			Module 5	5	
Block 4			Bridlington	14 } → 1	
Block 5			Module 6		
Psychiatry			Psychiatry		
Obstetrics			Module 7		
Aysgarth	36		Obstetrics		
Block 6			Annual leave		
Annual leave			(1 week)		
(4 weeks)			Module 8	5 } → 1	
Block 7			Biggleswade	20	
Aberdeen	6		Annual leave		
Ambleside	34		(2 weeks)		
Accident &			Module 9	16 } → 1	
emergency			Balmoral	34	
Amersham	2		Module 10	11 } → 1	
Arundel	2		Blackburn		
Block 8			Senior nursing		
Annual leave			module	4	
(4 weeks)			Theatre		
Block 9	2 } → 1		Braintree		
Aldeburgh	31		Barking	24	
Annual leave			Management		
(2 weeks)			module 1		
Balancing			Annual leave		
modules 1–5			(2 weeks)		
Ashington	9		Bromley	11 } → 1	
			Management		
			module 2	5	
Total score		5	Total score		12

The new scoring system turns out to make very little difference (see Table 11.19). The final scores still show the same relation: Hospitals 1 and 3 with almost identical scores, although Hospital 3 was more variable, and each of them was a long way below Hospital 2 (see Table 11.20).

In running an apprenticeship system of training, it is often quite difficult to know how well professed aims are being realised. The

259

Table 11.19: Estimate of uptake

Hospital 1		Hospital 2		Hospital 3	
Nurse	Score	Nurse	Score	Nurse	Score
101	37	201	105	301	49
103	36	203	115	303	46
105	40	205	81	305	30
107	42	207	101	307	46
109	42	209	97	309	33
111	37	211	76	311	36
113	43	213	104	313	38
115	45	215	110	315	47
117	40	217	104	317	32
119	40	219	103	319	40
121	41	221	79		
123	34	223	105		
125	39	225	100		
		227	79		
		229	94		
		231	121		
		233	98		

Mean: $\bar{x} = 39.7$
Standard deviation:
$s = 3.07$

Mean: $\bar{x} = 98.4$
Standard deviation:
$s = 12.94$

Mean: $\bar{x} = 39.7$
Standard deviation:
$s = 6.95$

Table 11.20: Average scores

Hospital 1, $\bar{x} = 39.7$	$s = 3.07$	(modified modular)
Hospital 2, $\bar{x} = 98.4$	$s = 12.94$	(modular)
Hospital 3, $\bar{x} = 39.7$	$s = 6.95$	(block)

results seem to indicate that Hospital 2 is achieving that integration of theory and practice desired by the proponents of the modular system.

Maximum possible scores and efficiency

By assuming that ward allocation is literally perfect, it is possible to calculate a maximum possible score for each training school for the given programme of classroom instruction. It is assumed that a perfect ward allocation scheme would enable each element of theory to be related contiguously and proportionately to clinical experience. Detailed calculation results in the following scores for each training scheme: in Hospital 1 : 192; in Hospital 2 : 278; in Hospital 3 : 148. The maxima are exactly in the order that one would expect: 'modular' highest; 'modified modular' second; and 'block' lowest.

It will be recalled that average integration scores were: Hospital 1, 39.7; Hospital 2, 98.4; and Hospital 3, 39.7. An estimate of *efficiency* of uptake can be made: Hospital 1, 20.7% (39.7/192); Hospital 2, 35.4% (98.4/278); and Hospital 3, 26.8% (39.7/148).

Hospital 2 achieves its high score in two ways: (1) the highest maximum; and (2) the highest percentage of this maximum. This suggests great care in both original course design and in the detail of ward allocation.

DISCUSSION

We turn now to implications and applications, to the ways in which staff of school and hospital can improve training by using the procedures outlined in this paper.

(1) The constraints of research

As researchers we were outsiders, with only a limited knowledge of each of the three local situations. A tutor, ward sister or nursing officer within any one of the three hospitals would have a greater and more subtle degree of knowledge of her particular milieu, deriving from a continuous intimacy with the institution. Also our purpose was general understanding rather than particular application, so that, for example, our clinical categorisation was necessarily rather coarse since it had to apply to all three hospitals.

(2) Setting up a monitoring system

Schools are becoming increasingly responsible for their own examination and training systems. Autonomy has its burdens, but these are eased by knowledge, and a better system for monitoring students would help substantially.

At the heart of our analysis is the classification of elements in both school and ward, leading finally to a composite set of clinical categories. For the purposes of a single hospital such a composite set could be designed by a group of staff selected from wards, senior nursing staff, and tutors. All the detail of local knowledge could be incorporated to produce a set of clinical categories closely tailored to the practice and needs of that particular institution.

261

Our categorisation was based on a medical model, because this was most appropriate for the three hospitals taken together; but our analysis is not dependent on this. A more nursing-oriented model of hospital treatment could be categorised and analysed similarly.

One could follow the procedures outlined in this chapter and calculate a set of integration scores for each student. The simple scoring system could be used, since we have shown that there seems to be little gain from using the more complex one. The records already exist to make this a fairly simple operation. It would not be essential to use a computer — we did not use one in our analysis — but for repeated application this would be the easiest way to proceed. The programme would be simple to write and, once in operation, the cost in time and resources would be negligible. Similar methods could be used to generate scores for assessing variety and extent of clinical opportunity (see Lewin and Jacka, 1985).

Meticulous planning is laborious, and to work within such a plan is constraining. An accurate monitoring system allied to a simple and approximate plan will achieve the same end more easily and less painfully. This is a cybernetic approach (in plain English: adjust as you go).

(3) Using a monitoring system

The pervasive effect of a monitoring system, once established, would derive from the increased precision of information available to tutorial staff about the educational progress of each student, and consequently about the training scheme in general. There would also be various particular uses of the monitoring information. We give two examples:

(a) Benchmarks. An accumulation of individual scores would enable one to set benchmarks which could be used as guides to acceptable levels of training.

(b) Allocation. The tutor could review the levels of clinical opportunity accumulated by a given student, some time in the latter part of her training. If in any area there were a substantial shortfall, this could be adjusted by a change in allocation, the student being placed on wards where the shortfall would be made up.

CONCLUSION

We have presented and analysed those parts of the Clinical Learning Project concerned with what we have described as academic and clinical opportunity, i.e. with the learning material available to the student nurses (school course content, and the stable pattern of clinical conditions on each ward). We have shown how, by observing and counting, and using only the simplest methods, one can construct coherent and illuminating *measures* of instruction, opportunity and integration in student nurse training. Finally, we have indicated how the tutorial staff of a training school could use the procedures of this chapter to devise a system for monitoring some aspects of the educational progress of their students.

REFERENCES

Georgopoulos, B.S. and Jackson, M.M. (1970) Nursing Kardex behaviour in an experimental study of patient units with and without clinical nurse specialists. *Nursing Research 19* (3), 196–218

Healy, E. and McGork, W. (1966) Effectiveness and acceptance of nurses' notes. *Nursing Outlook, 14* (3), 32–4

Leach, J. and Lewin, D.C. (1981) *The Clinical Learning Project: a study of the factors influencing the clinical learning of student nurses.* Nursing Education Research Unit, Chelsea College, University of London

Lelean, S. (1973) *Ready for report nurse?* Royal College of Nursing, London, pp. 105, 121

Lewin, D.C. and Jacka, K. (1985) *The clinical learning of student nurses; Part I: curriculum.* Nursing Education Research Unit, King's College (Chelsea), University of London

Roper, N. (1976) *Clinical experience in nurse education.* Churchill Livingstone, Edinburgh

Selmanoff, E.D. and Walker, V.H. (1964) A study of the nature and uses of nurses' notes. *Nursing Research, 13* (2), 113–31

Index